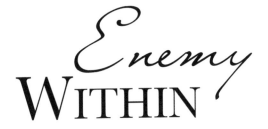

Enemy WITHIN

*A memoir of strength,
determination & acceptance*

KAREN AGER

NEW
HOLLAND

Dedicated

with all my love to Mum, Dad and Steve

In memory of

Peter and Jasmine Wells

Contents

Chapter 1	Life's a Beach	11
Chapter 2	Devil Inside	21
Chapter 3	Reason to Believe	35
Chapter 4	Horror Movie	50
Chapter 5	Back in Black	66
Chapter 6	Darling of the Universe	80
Chapter 7	Slipping Through my Fingers	97
Chapter 8	Weather With You	107
Chapter 9	Beautiful Day	118
Chapter 10	Empire State of Mind	132
Chapter 11	Handbags and Gladrags	143
Chapter 12	Angel On My Shoulder	159
Chapter 13	Melting Pot	172
Chapter 14	Comfortably Numb	185
Chapter 15	A Brave New World	198
Chapter 16	By Your Side	210
Chapter 17	Forever Young	223

Acknowledgements

Johanna Ager, my mother, I love you. You raised me to be resilient and determined. They're the qualities that I have always seen and admired in you. When you turned 70 you put your high heels on and took your black convertible for a spin; you have such a great spirit. Your positive, high energy, 'I Can' attitude is what I cherish about you and about our time together. Thanks for reminding me about how to have fun even when times were tough and for *always* being there. I look forward to champagne in Mornington.

My father, Max Ager, deserves credit for the wisdom in this book. You don't say a whole lot, Dad, but when you do your words are carefully chosen, insightful and smart. I admire your intellect and love your accidental humour.

To my big brother, Steve, you are my rock. I am so full of admiration for you and what you have achieved in your life. Thank you for giving me your blessing to write about our family. I know how proud you are and how hard it has been for you to let me 'hang all our family's dirty washing on the line.' But you knew I needed to write this and trusted me that it would be done in an authentic way to help and inspire others. I see the man you are—the wonderful brother, son, husband and father. Then I see the airline captain of the A380 and I am just in awe. I love you so much.

Matt, I'll be able to cook you dinner and be a 'proper wife' now that I'm finished the book. Thanks for doing all the little extra things around the house and for walking Willy when I couldn't. You helped me come up with words and sentences when I was too tired to think and supported me on this sometimes lonely journey. When I asked if I could share intimate details about our life together as husband and wife and your personal heartaches, you were generous and understood why they were important to my story. I look forward to growing old together. Thank you for finding the courage to work through your pain so that our marriage could have another chance. You are the love of my life. Willy, you have filled a void for both of us and helped heal our pain. I look forward to seeing your wagging tail every morning when I wake up.

Lisa, thank you for carrying my bags all around the world and for making me laugh when I was crying. You're the best friend I could have ever wished for. Uncle Jack, you lugged me up and down stairs and are the most selfless person I know. Thank you to the Readings for your lifelong friendship.

To my sisters-in-law, Trudy and Charlotte, your journeys have been tough. You are both incredibly courageous women, wonderful mothers to your sons and very special to me.

Father Michael Elligate, I am eternally grateful that you have been my spiritual guide throughout my journey with RA. Thank you.

To my friend Venessa, I admire you. It has become clearer to me in recent years that our friendship will be deep and everlasting and that our paths were meant to cross. You're one of the people I most like to spend time with because of the depth of your character and your endless spirit. Thanks for your support with the book...you know what I mean.

When I met John Singleton he had cancelled all scheduled meetings because his day wasn't going so well, but he still met with me. You read my book proposal and made a decision about whether to support it within a few days. You said, 'I get people pitching things all the time. I like to try to give one in ten young Australians a chance.' I was fortunate to see how you work and how you make successful decisions. Now I understand why you are such a successful man. Thanks for giving me that chance, Singo, and for picking up the phone and calling Kevin Weldon and Pam Seaborn.

On a cool July day I met with Kevin Weldon at Bondi Icebergs for lunch. We talked about aeroplanes and books. Thank you, Kevin, for supporting me and for your time. I am indebted to Pam Seaborn, my literary agent, for believing in this project and for taking me under her wing. I appreciate all your hard work and your graceful professionalism. Joan Stanbury edited my story and became my 'life coach' in the process. Thank you, Joan, for helping me believe in my ability to write, for telling me to 'just keep going', for your intellect and patience. To Fiona Schultz at New Holland, you had faith in my book when others didn't; for that I will always be grateful. I would also like to thank Diane Jardine at New Holland for having the patience of a saint.

Thank you to Pamela Marin who worked with me on the proposal. Suzanne Gleason, you gave me your time as we drank champagne and talked about my ideas for the book. You helped me to believe I could do this. You are great!

While I was in the final stages of editing the manuscript Ron Silver died. The news saddened me a great deal. Although we hadn't seen each other in years, I will always be grateful to him for planting the seed about my move to New York. Ron was an eloquent and gracious man and a good friend.

To the millions of people around the world who are suffering from arthritis and other chronic diseases this book is for you. Together we have a collective voice and together we can find a cure. We must *all* continue to have hope.

Dr Paula Marchetta, you once said I was one of your sickest patients. But you got me back on my feet. Thank you for your tender loving care and for your endless gentle words of encouragement.

Thank you to Jeffrey Gottfurcht and the dream board for inspiring me beyond the book. I look forward to making many dreams come true for children living with RA all over the world.

I would not have survived my life's journey without the following people to whom I will be eternally grateful. Thank you: DBD-David Pearlman, Tracey Moore, Vicky Semmel, Kelly Nixon, Uncle John Fikkers, my dear nephews, the Readings, Robbie Anthony, Trish Brennan, Lorraine Stephenson, Al Merrin (for answering all my desperate texts), Mark Lizotte (for the use of your lyrics and for singing my wedding song), Joseph Lebowitz and his wonderful family, the Mourlots, Laura Light, George Dymond, Linda Miglierina, Amy Iamundo and my UNIS family, Tony Moore, Jay Alger, Steve Terzuoli, Michael Friedman, Fiona Scott-Hanley, Seth Ginsberg, AARDA, AF, Jesica Church and so many more…

Foreword

In *Enemy Within,* Karen Ager tells a story which has desperately needed to be told. For the 46 million adults in the USA living with some form of arthritis, Karen's story will bring this hidden disease into public consciousness. With numbers estimated to rise to 67 million by the year 2030, Karen's memoir holds an important message of hope for sufferers.

Rheumatoid arthritis (RA) is the most crippling form of the disease and affects 3 million adults and 2 to 3 times more women than men. Few of us—even the doctors who care every day for patients suffering with RA—truly understand what it is like to live with the pain, limitation and isolation this disease causes. Few of us are aware of the profound effect the diagnosis of RA has on someone's life: on their future hopes, dreams and even the very scope of what may or may not be possible to do in the routine business of everyday living. Karen gives us a moving view of that inner world. Afflicted with severe RA as a teenager, she is robbed of the carefree joys of adolescence and struggles to come to terms with a disease which will never leave her and for which treatments have been neither fully adequate, nor safe. With amazing spirit, Karen finds her way, pulling herself up from the dark despair of disability imposed by her disease. Through the recounting of her life with RA, we see how Karen has learned to triumph, not despite her disease, but because of it.

What becomes clear as you read this book is that Karen has grown into such a remarkable woman because of the very disease which she has fought against so hard. Eventually, her assiduous efforts to hide the shame of her affliction and be 'normal' give way to a growing determination to become an advocate for others who also suffer, often alone and in silence. By telling her story, Karen gives those with RA a beautiful and heartfelt voice which inspires hope and inspiration.

RA has robbed Karen of many things, but it has also given her incredible courage, perseverance, resilience and a rare appreciation for the simple joys of life, no matter what difficulties must be faced. It is said that you do not get porcelain unless you go through the white heat of the kiln. You will see in reading Karen's story that her spirit shines, with a richness and luster only found in the finest porcelain.

Paula Marchetta, MD, MBA
New York

Chapter 1
Life's a Beach

I was on my beach—Black Rock on Melbourne's Port Phillip Bay—on a blistering summer afternoon, watching my cousin, David, jog to the water's edge. He high-stepped like a gazelle through the shallows and then executed a perfect swallow-dive into the bay.

Beach days in Australia are like beach days in many other parts of the world. It could have been the Hamptons, New York or Venice Beach, California. The teenage energy was the same—out of control hormones, slim athletic bodies, the hope of finding true love and *the scene*. Girls are chasing lifeguards, there's experimentation with drinking and smoking, music pumps and there are acres of naked skin.

Lazing around on the sand I stared at the familiar sight of the Red Bluff cliffs extending into the bay. The gently lapping waves licked the custard-yellow sand. The guys from the local private schools began arriving on the beach. They threw off their shirts to reveal young, perfect chests as they raced each other to the water. I began to squirm on my towel hoping that none of them would see me and decide to pay me a visit. I rolled over and hid my face in the cups of my hands. Sweat bubbled on my forehead, but I didn't care, I just didn't want to be seen. This was part of the reason I preferred to go to Black Rock beach *without* my girlfriends. They attracted attention.

I had two groups of schoolmates. Jackie was the *glamourpuss* amongst us. She was blonde, sporty and had a figure to die for. Her mum gave her the freedom to do what she wanted and her confidence attracted what we considered the *coolest* guys. When I went to the beach with

Jackie we were never alone for long. I didn't like it—there was no way I could relax.

My other group of friends were of a more academic bent— lawyers-in-the-making. They chose to study rather than hang out with their less-serious fellow students and even in the late 1970s were sensible enough to stay out of the sun. One of them, Helen, had set her sights on being named dux of Mentone Girls' High School and we all just accepted that it would happen. She was pretty with short brown hair, and I thought she worried about the size of her large breasts too much. Perhaps I was envious. Sandra, another academic friend, was cute and quirky. We'd all get together at street parties once in a while.

These friendships offered meaning to my life at a time when everything else seemed to be falling apart. Together we shared our teenage hopes and dreams about the future. I loved the contrast of values between my two groups of friends. The challenge of trying to corrupt Helen and Sandra by exposing Jackie's daredevil exploits tossed a healthy dose of comedy into the mix.

My cousin David had come from Sydney to stay with us during the holidays and we had walked to Black Rock beach together. When he burst through the water with a flick of his sleek brown hair, I flipped on to my stomach and began fiddling with the pages of *Dolly* magazine that were smeared with suntan oil. Reading about the next Dolly Cover Girl didn't interest me much, nor did the 'Are you trying to be popular?' quiz. I just wanted to be out there, swimming with David, matching his strokes as he swam to the rusting *Cerberus* battleship. Its wrecked remains protruded in the distance from the glassy bay.

The *Cerberus* had been scuttled in 1926 by the Royal Australian Navy. Its half-submerged hull had become a breakwater, defending beachgoers from waves whipped up when Melbourne's changeable weather turned foul. It was also a swim-dare destination for us local kids.

At 15 and already as tall as Mum, I was a strong swimmer. I could have kept up with my cousin in Port Phillip Bay, but I wasn't keen on making the short hike across soft, uneven sand to the water.

There was also the matter of my pink-flowered bikini top. I wished it had more to cover. A recent growth spurt had taken me up over the heads of most of my classmates, but other girls my age were growing in ways that interested the boys more. And then there was my coordination—or lack of it. I was known for tripping and falling, for missing chairs when I tried to sit and letting plates and cups slip from my hands.

Still, I might have risked 50 paces through shifting sand in a bikini, even with those pompous, private school boys tossing a football nearby, eyeing the girls like hungry gulls. But darker worries pinned me to my towel.

To an outsider looking in we were the perfect family—my airline pilot father, my glamorous mother, my tall, handsome brother and me. In reality, all was far from well.

Within the walls of our immaculate home my parents' marriage was crumbling and my brother and I, though calm and resilient on the surface, were caught up in undercurrents of tension and insecurity.

With David as a house guest for our New Year celebrations, my family had papered over all the problems and put on a 'no-worries' facade—but he was due to leave in a few days. My brother, Steve, would soon be studying full-time to become a pilot at the local flying school. He planned to begin his course in January. With our parents' marriage floundering, Steve was my rock. I had so many fears for the future, but the most pressing one was that I didn't know how I was going to continue fitting into life at home when the foundations were so rocky.

After we moved into our new house in the Melbourne bayside suburb of Black Rock—a custom-built, stylishly decorated showplace that Mum kept spotless—I became aware that the glue that had held my parents together was becoming unstuck. Or maybe there had been problems in their marriage from the start. Evidence of the friction between them came to me as I lay under my lime, daisy-covered duvet in bed. The brick wall behind my headboard went down to the rumpus room, where Mum and Dad convened for drinks and arguments. Their voices floated through to my room with disturbing clarity.

Sometimes they squabbled about my father's pastimes. As a captain with Trans Australia Airlines (TAA), Dad was often away on interstate flights. I remember he was away 14 Christmases in a row. As a child, my clearest memory of Dad was of him smartly dressed in his uniform, cap and all, leaving as we waved goodbye to him from our front porch. Somehow he still found time to build a sailing boat in our garage, a project Mum hated for its mess. Later on Dad fancied himself as a gold prospector and busily researched abandoned mines and ordered gold-detecting machinery from America. To Mum, whose Dutch parents left war-ravaged Holland with eight children in tow, Dad's hobbies were over the top and she considered them nothing more than childish indulgences.

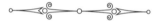

Mum and her family arrived in Australia in August 1950. Slots were filling up quickly at the Bathurst Holding Centre (migrant camp) as displaced Europeans fled their home countries. Australia believed it must populate or perish. Because of the huge numbers of immigrants arriving on its shores, within a few generations Australia changed from an Anglo-Celtic population to a multicultural one.

Mum was just one of two million post-war arrivals. As her family tried to settle into the camp, there were already signs of overcrowding. Existing army barracks had filled up and acres of khaki canvas were being used in the construction of a temporary tent city. Clattering pots boomed from the communal kitchens and broken English conversations echoed from the bathrooms. Mum sat on the side of her steel-framed bed and sobbed.

'*Ik wil terug naar Nederland, terug naar mijn school in Groningen…*'

'I want to go back to The Netherlands, back to my school in Groningen,' she cried.

Everything in Australia was so different from the Dutch landscape and way of life. The change to her life was fundamental. She was no longer Anneke, she was Johanna. She was no longer Dutch, she was 'New Australian' (the term coined in one of Australia's first attempts at political correctness—it replaced the derogatory-sounding *Reffos*, short for refugees).

My mother's very identity had been stripped from her and in the ultimate humiliation she had no real address, just a number in a holding centre camp. Her tears were the same as the tears of every other child there; they needed a home not just a roof over their heads. She was grieving for everything that had been familiar—even the security of her snowy walk to school on well-worn, uncomfortable cobbled streets.

Eventually Mum was sent to work at the age of 14 because her family had little money. Determined to achieve, she worked her way up from clipping cottons at a garment factory in Wollongong to modelling the clothes that her fellow workers made. On the catwalk she was a very impressive figure and before long she was approached to enter the Miss Australia Quest. Her confidence was growing but, with a Dutch-speaking family at home, her English lagged behind. Passing up the opportunity to enter the quest she worked overtime to improve her English-language skills and in the early 1960s travelled to Sydney to become an air hostess in the still-glamorous world of flight. It was a sure-fire route to matrimony.

Mum began flying with East West Airlines, a regional carrier in New South Wales. She met my father when, as a potential tenant, she visited his apartment in the sun-drenched eastern Sydney suburb of Bondi.

Bondi is at the heart of a magical coastline of curling beaches, headlands with cascading cliffs and an ocean that never ends. It is a place for summer romances and midnight skinny dips. For decades, airline pilots have met and fallen in love with air hostesses—now called, less romantically, 'flight attendants'—on its glistening sands.

Bondi, meaning 'sounds of water breaking on the beach', is beautiful—but the beauty can hide treachery. Well known for its surf and strong currents, in 1938 freak waves swept 300 bathers from a sandbank into a rip which took them out to sea. Eighty Bondi lifesavers rescued all but five swimmers. The day became known as Black Sunday to the locals.

Dad's apartment backed right on to Bondi beach. A leap over the fence and he'd be in the surf.

Mum's Catholic upbringing clashed with her natural instincts so she wasn't much into dating. Dad had immediately fallen in love with this beautiful *New Australian* Catholic girl with Grace Kelly looks. After a lightning courtship they became engaged and were married soon afterwards.

Cast out of the workforce at 22 because of her marital status, Mum embraced her new family life with enthusiasm. With the work ethic of her Dutch heritage, she slaved, non-stop, to make a good home for her young husband. After just a year of marriage she fell pregnant with my brother Steve. The birth of her beautiful baby boy brought tension to the marriage, but Mum was an adoring mother and tried her best to support her husband in his flying career.

Two and half years and a miscarriage later I was born. A blue-eyed, blonde-haired daughter. I was the apple of my father's eye. Six weeks after my birth, Dad was transferred to Port Moresby, Papua New Guinea (PNG). It was to be our home for the next four years. In the 1960s New Guinea was not a very safe place—for living or for flying. A geologically young country, its mountains are high, rugged and not always well-mapped; the oceans surrounding it are dangerously deep and airstrips are short, often angled and buffeted by winds that come from every which-way. The landing strips always seem to run directly into hills.

Dad went away for week-long trips and the very thought of leaving his wife and young family behind in a compound—surrounded by high security fences—made him physically ill.

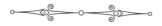

Dad was born in Melbourne in 1936, during the Great Depression. Two years earlier, in the city's centenary year, a third of Melbourne's population had lost their jobs and there was violence in the city's streets. Despite being raised in such difficult times his mother nurtured in him a love of planes. A few decades later my mother would do the same for her son.

Tall and skinny, Dad was bullied at school for being too smart. A loner, he pedalled 19 miles from his home to watch light aircraft take off and land at Essendon Aerodrome, an airport made famous by the aviation pioneer Sir Charles Kingsford Smith in the 1920s and by the arrival of the Beatles in June 1964. For Dad, watching the planes take off and land at the airport was the perfect escape. It was his favourite place to be. These stolen moments at Essendon paved the way for his aviation career. He got to know the workers there and when he left school at the age of 16, he landed a job overhauling aircraft engines. It didn't matter to Dad that the hangar was cold and dirty and a persistent draught gusted under the gap between the concrete floor and the gray, steel pulley door. Thirty shillings was the pay for a week's work. The job came with one huge advantage—it gave Dad the opportunity to learn to fly. After 40 hours of work he was entitled to a one-hour flying lesson. It was a perfect scenario for a solitary boy who loved planes.

After receiving an enviable 100 per cent pass mark for most of his flying examinations, he was interviewed for a job at TAA—dressed in his father's dark suit, the only one in the family—and later became one of the airline's youngest captains.

A second-generation Aussie with English Methodist roots, Dad converted to the Catholic faith to marry Mum but rarely came to mass at St Brigid's. He also didn't hide his dislike of all things Catholic—especially nuns. As I lay under my daisy duvet, I often heard derogatory remarks about the Church and the Brigidine Sisters.

'I don't want them ruining Karen,' Dad would spit at Mum in a voice lubricated by a couple of whiskies.

'What do you mean—ruining?' my mother would shoot back.

I could picture Mum sitting primly at the red leather bar, a long-stemmed wine glass in her hand.

'I want her to get a proper education,' she would counter.

Dad would storm: 'She can get a proper education in a state school—*just like I did*. And she won't ruin her sex life listening to some crazy nun.'

Sex: that was the rub. A year before, Mum had met another man who had taken a keen interest in her. Dad found out. One night

I overheard them arguing about a bank account my mother had opened in Perth, on Australia's west coast.

'That's where he lives, isn't it?' Dad accused her. His voice, transmitted to my room upstairs, was loud and rough.

I knew Mum was keen on Perth. The month before she'd dragged my brother and me across the continent to stay in a fancy hotel there. She was scouting *her* new life, saying how good it would be for *us*.

Perth! The loneliest city on earth! Two thousand miles from Black Rock!

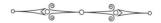

Frying on my beach towel that day on Black Rock beach, I bristled with rage. I tossed aside *Dolly*, fed up with everything and everyone, including or maybe especially those curvy magazine models bursting from their bikinis.

A shadow fell across my towel. David. Back from his swim. He shook his head like a terrier, dousing me with cold beads of sea water.

'Hey!' I said, laughing, but as I tried to squirm away I felt a sharp stab on my right side. It felt like a hot dagger had been thrust into my flesh. It seemed to grind and twist into my hip. My joint throbbed. Had I somehow pulled a muscle? I fell back on the beach towel. David smiled at me. He must have thought I was playing around as I held my side and gasped for breath.

'C'mon, Kaz,' he said, using my nickname. 'It's time to go.'

'Hang on,' I said, trying to be brave, trying to breathe. I tried to push myself up but that made the pain worse and, though I would have given anything not to cry, my eyes filled with tears. All I could think of was what would my handsome cousin—on whom I had a not-so-secret crush—would think of me now?

'What's the matter with you?' He knelt beside me.

'I can't get up. I must have pulled a muscle in my leg.'

My burly six-foot-three-inch-tall cousin smiled, shrugged his wide shoulders, scooped me up and carried me home.

This wasn't a pulled muscle; it was my disease, introducing itself to me. It was a warning that I was under attack. A war for my body had started—only I didn't know it. The opposing sides in the battle that was going on within had been assembled and were ready to march towards the front-line. Shots were fired and my hip was assaulted. But we were all too ignorant to know what was happening and I was too ignorant to listen to my body.

David carried me home. Mum put me to bed with a kiss and an aspirin. In the morning I felt fine, the memory of yesterday's scare dissolved like a dream.

One thing remained. The stress of Mum and Dad's failing marriage and the guilt I took on board because of it became a breeding ground for my disease. It was just what it needed. It began to fester, like some perverse cold sore that takes over perfectly shaped lips and deforms them. We had no idea of the power of rheumatoid arthritis to permanently reshape fingers to bulbous, bent twigs like those of an evil witch. Nothing was further from our minds. My body was about to embark on a lifelong fight with itself and I, along with my family, was absolutely oblivious to it all.

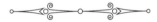

A little more than a year after the Black Rock beach assault on my hip I awoke, at home, to find I couldn't get out of bed. My fingers were so swollen I couldn't grasp the duvet. My wrists were so weak I couldn't push myself up. And there was something wrong with my ankles, too. I couldn't move my feet.

'Mum! Dad! *Mum!*'

My parents were deeply worried.

Until then, perhaps because everyone was so preoccupied with their own problems or simply because none of us had ever been faced with a serious illness before, the enemy that was stalking me was ignored. There had been a string of incidents, but, as a family we just accepted each one as it happened and didn't think seriously about any of them.

I couldn't unload the dishwasher without a glass or plate slipping through my fingers and smashing on the floor. 'For God's sakes,'

Dad would mutter, heading for the broom closet.

On holiday in Portsea—a chic, upmarket sea-side resort village close to the point where Melbourne's Port Phillip Bay meets the Southern Ocean—I fell down so many times it became a family joke.

'There she goes again,' I'd hear as my gangly legs, like those of a new-born colt, gave way yet again. I would end up on the floor in a tangled mess, limbs askew.

My parents shrugged, no doubt thinking I would grow out of my physical ineptitudes.

'She's going through a phase', my mother would say.

My friends thought I was a bit clumsy, but we girls had more important concerns, like the latest beauty tips in *Dolly* magazine. So I got on with it. In Australia, we do tend to get on with things—we ignore problems or discuss them with our friends rather than see a doctor or stretch out on a couch and spill the beans to a psychoanalyst. The widespread view is: if you have a friend, who needs a 'shrink'? 'She'll be right, mate!'

Chapter 2
Devil Inside

Instead of Perth, Mum moved to the back bedroom. She and Dad still rumbled in the rumpus room now and then and sometimes he stole to her bedside with a flashlight hours later, waking her with a blast of light so they could continue their row.

I was into adolescence and into the driver's seat. Dragging myself over the hills on my red Malvern Star bicycle, I'd watch all the other kids ride past me eager to get home after school. Balcombe Road, on the route home, seemed to get longer and the inclines steeper every day.

For me it felt like a balancing act—at home and on my bike. I juggled balancing myself and my overloaded school bag as I stood to find the extra power in my legs to pedal to the top of the hill. But what did I care? I wasn't in a rush. I hated going home anyway. Always late, I'd glide down the pebbled driveway dragging my feet to make skid marks in the gravel just because Mum hated me doing that. I stood at the front door of our brand new Black Rock house, staring at the keyhole. As I slid the key into the silver lock, a surge of anger would rise, almost automatically. I never knew which gear to slip into before facing my family. Would they be arguing tonight or would we be in *happy family* mode? Turning the key to unlatch the door was like opening a jack-in-the-box. I could never be sure what to expect. So I would cower inside, eat a 'truckload of biscuits' just because my mother hated it. She said it would spoil my dinner. I'd refuse to talk about my day, then retreat to the safe haven of my bedroom and cry.

Steve's room was next to mine. With my brother studying to be a pilot, he was absent a lot. I'd treasure the times we were together in his room. It was filled with good memories—model airplanes, miniature thatched Fijian bures bought at markets on past holidays and numerous Herald Premiership posters depicting the Hawthorn Football Club's golden era in the 1970s.

Sometimes I'd pester Steve and sit, leaning against his bed, knees scrunched to my chest, toes rubbing on the shag pile carpet. He'd always make me laugh and I'd believe, at least for the moment, that things were going to work out for our family. Mostly though, I felt alone, lost in the remains of my parents' scuttled marriage. I didn't know who to turn to. Mum, with her perfect looks, perfect house, perfect handmade clothes and perfect poise with strangers, or Cruisin' Dad, who was now taking holidays alone to the Pacific Islands and dressing as Fred Flintstone on ships' fancy dress nights.

Whoever I chose would be wrong. It hurt me to have to choose. I loved them both. But one thing was for sure, the umbrella of pretence under which we were all living as 'the perfect family' would soon be over. It had to be. The stress was too much for us all.

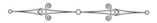

Mum had always spoken about the pride one feels from having a job so I decided I would give it a try. As soon as I turned 16 I took a part-time job at a Mentone grocery store. On Fridays and Saturdays I was a 'check-out chick' in a yellow apron, standing for long shifts that often netted me puffy ankles and sore knees. My discomfort was dismissed by my family as 'growing pains' and I learned to ease the agony with long, hot showers. I liked having my own money—and getting out of that damned house.

One Friday night I stepped into the Black Rock house still wearing my yellow apron to a chorus of 'Surprise!'. Mum had secretly invited friends to mark my seventeenth birthday with sausage rolls and a birthday cake. Though I smiled and chatted like a trouper I was furious. What a pretence, I thought. I was sick of play-acting the role of dutiful daughter in a happy, loving family.

That night I met Geoff who, though uninvited, had come to the party with a mate. Tall, dark and with a body that was finely tuned from the sport he played, Geoff belonged to the highly ranked St Kilda professional football team, which in the 1990s became a part of the fast-expanding Australian Football League (AFL). When he asked if he could call me, I was thrilled. Over the next few weeks he pursued me relentlessly and eventually became my first boyfriend. He was a welcome respite from the pain that engulfed my family life.

Not long after my birthday party my mother decided she had endured enough of her sham marriage. Again she made plans to go to Perth to join the man who, for some years, had wanted her in his life. The move to the back bedroom had just amplified the tension in the house. I didn't know it at the time, but we had only a few months left as a 'real' family. By October 1981, I would have finished my Higher School Certificate (HSC) and Steve was already in flying school. Mum thought her responsibilities to her children were almost over so she made preparations to leave.

I didn't fully understand all of Mum's reasons for wanting to go so far away from her children. I knew her health was not the best—she had undergone three operations for kidney stones—and that we were all suffering from living together in a house that was overloaded with stress because of my parents' arguments. But that's all I really comprehended.

As one of eight children, Mum came from a family where decisions were made by her parents and were not discussed with her or her siblings. As the second eldest, she was always just told what she had to do. As a mother herself, I think she figured she would keep Steve and me protected for as long as she could by isolating us from her troubles. She maintained a facade that all was well, while tossing her problems over and over in her mind, desperately seeking a solution. She completely overlooked the fact that 'D-day' would come eventually. She didn't understand that when this day arrived, her decision was a huge shock to us all. Her failure to discuss the problem from the start just aggravated the situation and intensified everybody's emotions.

Steve and I knew about her plans to move to Perth a few weeks in advance. Dad didn't have the luxury of this warning. Steve understood better than me that Mum's health was at risk so he supported her, accepted her decision to leave and got on with it. I just got angry. I also began to feel responsible for her unhappiness and guilty because I was the 'difficult daughter' she never thought she'd have. The difference between how Steve and I handled things was more marked as the days passed. But as guilty as I felt about Mum, I still knew in my heart that there was something innately wrong about her decision to move so far away from my brother and me. In my heart I felt betrayed, yet I never told my father of her plan to leave.

I stood on the well-groomed gravel driveway that I'd so liked to spoil and waved her farewell. Her silver Celica was packed to the brim. She planned to drive to Adelaide and put herself, her car and her life on the Indian-Pacific railroad. This transcontinental train connects ocean to ocean, the east coast to the west coast, over miles of a harsh, barren plain known as the Nullarbor—meaning, literally, 'no trees'.

Although the shock of Mum leaving home didn't really impact me until later, the reality of her situation must have glared starkly back at her, crippling her mind as she travelled from one side of Australia to the other. It was a cruel, lonely reality that only the rugged Australian landscape can drive home. Fresh from school where we had learnt Australian history, my grim thoughts went to the early explorer Edward John Eyre. In a moment of miserable insight I considered the fact that he must have felt the same when he was the first to walk across the continent in 1841.

Dad's reality was pretty stark too. Strangely, I don't remember where Steve was the day Mum left. I do know that I waited alone until nightfall for Dad to return from his trip. I saw the headlights turn into the drive. His first hint of what was to come was the absence of her car in the garage. I wondered if he'd pick that up. Soon enough I heard him unlock the front door and call out 'Hi'. When he entered the house he found it emptied of all that made it feel like home. His wife had gone and so had the feminine touches that Mum had so liked to scatter around the place.

Dad and I sat and sobbed. I'd only ever seen him cry once; that was when Charlie died. Charlie was our pet corgi who was hit by a car because I had decided to walk him without a leash. There we sat, on the same brown velvet couch that had been the meeting point for many family celebrations and cried. Dad and I both knew their marriage was over for good this time. It took a while for me to appreciate the connection between Dad's tears for Mum and his tears for Charlie, the family dog. But in the end, I understood that his tears were about loss. They were about loving and losing. This was a pivotal moment in Dad's life, and it was a moment that would bond us forever because I caught a glimpse of his soul that night.

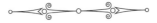

In 1982 I was 17, just out of high school and eager to start at a travel industry trade school. I had passed my HSC with impressive results despite family upsets and a three-month absence due to a bout of glandular fever that I just couldn't shake off. My whole family had been involved in the airline business, now it was my turn to spread my wings. To follow in their footsteps was all I ever desired. I did give one other vocation a fleeting thought—teaching might be an acceptable alternative. Fate was to play a decisive role.

One January morning the next assault of my disease happened. I woke with so many tender and swollen joints that I couldn't get out of bed. Ankles, knees, hips, fingers, wrists—every joint all the way up to my jaw—were sore. I was crippled. Disabled. Rigid. Pain bored deep within as I lay in my bed under my duvet cover. The mere thought of getting dressed exhausted me. Could I even make it from the bed to the cupboard to choose an outfit? Maybe I could drag myself? Did I have something to wear without buttons because my wrists were so swollen and I knew I wouldn't be able to put buttons through buttonholes. How would I make it down the stairs for breakfast? How could I eat breakfast when I couldn't raise my hand to my mouth because of my swollen elbows? Today even living was a chore. My pain dictated my mood. I was scared. I'd lost control of my body. I screamed, 'Mum, Muuuum, can you come here?' But Mum had gone.

I knew for the first time that my mother's love was no longer available at my beck and call and I had to accept that. So I lay there, crying, unable to move. I cried for hours that morning—alone in my room with my unwanted companion, my disease.

Even though my relationship with Mum was strained at times I knew in my heart if I asked for her help she'd be there for me. I telephoned her. Without hesitation, she flew back to Melbourne from Perth. I began to understand how hard it had been for her to leave me. Slowly we began to heal our relationship. It felt good. While she was home, together we sought answers from the medical profession.

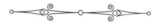

My local doctor referred me to a rheumatologist. I had little interest in acquainting myself with Dr Littlegeorge, especially when he put a name to my pains and physical ineptitude: Rheumatoid Arthritis (RA). The blood tests had revealed all. The doctor confirmed I had RA and then sombrely followed on with a pronunciation of the buzzwords of my disease: Progressive. Degenerative. Incurable.

Sometimes our long-term companions choose us, and we have little say in the matter. When the relationship is an abusive one, we may learn to shake them, take control, and move on. Other times, the union winds up being a lifelong one, and we learn to adapt, fight back and make the best of things. Rheumatoid arthritis would become my constant companion. It would be many years before I truly understood what those two words would mean to me. Within my body, a real war was taking shape and my oppressor was subtly moving forward readying itself for its campaign.

Nearly one in 5 Australians—that's 3.85 million—have arthritis, 46 million Americans and 350 million people worldwide have some form of the disease. Arthritis is a joint-stiffening disease usually thought of as an inevitable byproduct of the aging process. Rheumatoid Arthritis (RA) is its wicked, more virulent cousin. It's an autoimmune disease, like AIDS, that causes one's body to attack itself. It is chronic, progressive, deforming and as yet incurable. RA wreaks havoc with the joints, causing painful flare-ups and loss of mobility. Its primary target is the musculoskeletal system, but it can also damage the heart, lungs and eyes. Researchers don't know if RA's source is viral or bacterial, whether genetics play a role, or if stress is part of the triggering mechanism. But whatever its origin, RA cripples, and it can kill. And the cyclical nature of its symptoms wreaks a different kind of havoc, deforming self-perception, damaging plans. For many RA sufferers like me, the disease begins almost invisibly, with occasional joint "flare-ups" and other subtle signs of the inner destruction that limits mobility and can lead to disfigurement, joint-replacement surgeries—even death.

On one level, it all began to come together. The pieces of the jigsaw that my family and I had eyed in isolation—and, at times, puzzlement—were put into place by Dr Littlegeorge. All the episodes of adolescent 'butter fingers', growing pains and inexplicable tumbles suddenly evolved into a full picture. As we listened to him I remembered the year all the girls at school wore gold bangles. I couldn't—my body had too much acidity the jeweller told me. He'd sold me a bangle and exchanged it twice, but the third time I returned it complaining that it was shedding gold flakes he diagnosed the problem as mine, not his.

On a more immediate level, I did what teenagers are programmed to do in matters of mortality, responsibility and the future. I blocked it out, numbed it with more immediate concerns and filed it away in an inaccessible place. The doctor said I had a disease with no cure, a disease that would almost certainly cripple me, but I chose to treat it as a minor inconvenience, like a bout of influenza.

Mum and I went down the steps of the old Victorian house in Melbourne where the rheumatologist had his surgery, climbed into my shiny, electric-blue Mazda and headed for home. The air was bright with summer sunshine—a perfect beach day. I rolled down my window to let the wind whip my lemon-juice-lightened blonde hair and fiddled with the radio until I found a song I liked, a new one by the American group Foreigner. Cranking up the volume I sang along…*I've been waiting…for a girl like you…to come into my life*. By my feet were pamphlets that the doctor had given us which described my disease and provided contacts for support groups—along with a 12-week supply of cortisone and anti-inflammatory drugs.

I closed my eyes, wishing I were with Geoff.

I had the medication. In my mind my problem was now taken care of. Mum packed her bags and flew home to Perth.

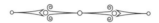

A few months earlier I'd been an inexperienced schoolgirl with a crush on a good-looking 'Aussie Rules' football player. The game, played with an egg-shaped ball, is—and always will be—the pride of Melburnians.

The sport began, unofficially, in 1858 when the Cambridge-educated Headmaster of Melbourne Grammar School suggested there be a masculine game played to keep his boys fit during the winter months. It evolved without rules, with bits taken from the many varied football traditions brought to Australia by convicts, colonizers and, later, British migrants.

To the casual and uninformed observer a game of Australian Rules football still looks like there are no rules. The players wear shorts that are Mardi Gras-tight and the sleeveless jumpers (jerseys), by design or accident, show off the players' biceps. Most sports seem to have phased out shiny polyester material but not Aussie Rules. The end result is an outfit that resembles that worn by the Bee Gees in the 'Staying Alive' video, crossed with John Travolta in *Saturday Night Fever* at a gay pride charity football match.

The Melbourne Cricket Ground (MCG) is the ideal stadium and backdrop for Aussie Rules. Meat pie-eating, beer-drinking spectators roar and scream at these fashion-conscious macho men of one team leaping high in the air to catch the ball and then kicking, running or hand-balling it down to their scoring end of the oval. Members of the opposing team tackle, punch and block them in an attempt to win the ball and, if successful, head back down to the other end of the oval to, hopefully, score through their own goal posts.

The players seem to feel a disproportionate amount of Australian pride in the game due, perhaps, to the lack of padded accessories under their sleeveless jumpers. Geoff was no exception.

What is also disproportionate is the widely felt Aussie sentiment that it is the toughest and best sport in the world. The Yanks think American Football is the best and the Brits think the same of soccer. We think our game is the best. Who knows and more importantly, does it really matter? Aussie males think it does. 'Football, meat pies, kangaroos and Holden cars' sums up the complete and very content Australian male. A 'sheila' for some drunken sex and to knock up breakfast the morning after is also good but not essential.

Now I had Geoff—my very own Aussie Rules football player. He'd pursued me relentlessly and I was proud he was my boyfriend. With Geoff I could escape into his football world and leave the pain of my world behind.

I really didn't know why my father scowled when he saw the yellow bumper sticker on Geoff's Holden station wagon: 'Save a mouse, eat a pussy'. To me, it was exciting—a dose of instant 'beach cred'. I knew Holden station wagons were called 'shaggin' wagons' because so many of them sported a mattress in the back and a surfboard on the racks.

Football was primarily a winter sport, while Australia's summer pop culture was all about the beach and surfing. It's the only continent in the world where nearly every town within cooee of a beach has a pub, a post office and a surf shop. The laid-back sport of surfing gave birth to the infamous 'no worries' attitude of Australians. It is what tea is to the English and what waving the Stars and Stripes is to an American. In many ways it defines us as a nation.

Geoff was a typical young Australian male. He was an Aussie Rules footballer with a surf board and a white Holden station wagon with a mattress in the back. He'd been trying to get me on it for weeks.

One cool night at the Sandringham drive-in theatre, as James Bond outmanoeuvred bad guys in *For Your Eyes Only*, Geoff manoeuvred me out of my virginity. I don't remember whether the earth moved, or much else about the event. What mattered to me was that I was the last of my group of girlfriends to have held on to her virginity and I was relieved to be rid of it. So that was sex and we returned to the front seat to see how James was getting on. Predictably, he was stuck in a pool of sharks again. His rocket-launcher pen leapt to the rescue.

The Sandringham drive-in served up yet another dose of popular Aussie culture. I'd grown up with drive-in cinemas—Mum and Dad in the front seat of the car, Steve and me, pyjama-clad and with pillows, in the back. The *Cinema of Distraction* (so-called by Ben Goldsmith) had certainly grown since its pre-World War II origins when cars were parked, facing a canvas hoisted between two gum trees, in a clearing on a farming property in Dunsborough, Western Australia.

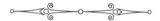

A few months after that infamous night, I began my year-long course at the William Angliss Travel and Tourism School in Melbourne. I was no longer a naïve, virginal schoolgirl and I was excited about beginning my travel career.

The commute was hard for me. Not because of the train rides, but because of the 20-minute walks from the train station to the school. Despite my new regimen of prescription pills, I woke most days with swollen ankles and knees and limped into the shower to let the hot water ease my pain. Overnight my knees would fill with fluid, making the skin surrounding the joints so tight I couldn't bend them. Stepping up into the shower was a problem. I'd hold on to the glass shower door and drag my legs up and over the one small step. My shoulders and wrists were also red, hot and swollen. Moving them even a centimetre was excruciatingly painful as they ground away, bone on bone.

While undertaking my formal classroom training for a job in the travel industry I did work experience at Qantas Airlines. My mother's work ethic must have rubbed off because I was considered conscientious and when my spell of work experience finished I was offered full-time shiftwork. Wooed by the prospect of a healthy income, I accepted the job and planned to continue going to school in my spare time.

None of it was what I'd hoped for.

My classes were dull and work meant eight-hour shifts of sitting in a booth with a telephone headset, tapping a keyboard. I was surrounded by a sea of cubicles filled with others all doing the same thing. It was called Airline Reservations. Not quite the same as the glamorous life of a flight attendant that I'd envisaged when I scribbled down 'travel industry' as my career choice in Year 9 at high school.

I was beginning to feel that RA was trying to beat me. I wasn't well enough to fly. My disease took care of that. The closest I got to becoming a 'flightie' was when Qantas managers dressed me up in a flight attendant's uniform to host an event. There I stood, wearing the 1980s floral colours of the company, meeting and greeting businessmen with a fake smile plastered on my face. The reality of working in the travel industry didn't match my dream of following in Mum's footsteps. I was overwhelmed by sadness. I was 19 and RA was stripping me of my childhood fantasies. In that uniform I felt like a phony.

Geoff was becoming a problem too, especially in the football off-season.

Success on the sporting field had boosted his ego and this, coupled with a lack of formal education and a difficult home life proved a volatile combination. He was very possessive and had violent mood swings that were fuelled by too much alcohol. An evening out would often end in a screaming argument with displays of physical aggression. He would punch walls, threaten other men if they spoke to me and subtly berate me with snide comments whispered in my ear. He was always quick to rise to the challenge of 'correcting' anyone, including myself, who would question his dominance over me.

If another male spoke to me he'd whisper: 'He wouldn't bother with you if he knew about your disease.'

My problem was that I was addicted to him. In my mind, I had *footballer wife status*—and with that went VIP treatment at games, free-flowing champagne at post-game parties and plenty of ego-boosting reflected glory. The scene was sweet, enticing and I desired it. However, the stress associated with living the high life triggered my RA to flare relentlessly, again and again. I'd wake most nights with crippling attacks that grew more and more frequent. My wrists began on a path of self-destruction, the bones fusing together so that they would no longer bend. The pain was excruciating; boring deeply into my joints. It felt like white ants gnawing within. Brushing my hair and teeth were quickly becoming impossible tasks for me. Still, I forced my aching limbs out of bed in the mornings even if I hobbled around like my grandmother. I just craved to be 'normal', and by denying that my disease existed I fooled myself into believing that it was true.

Despite all my efforts, deep down I felt I was changing. My disease was not only influencing my body but also my spirit. The pain was starting to impact every dimension of my life. Until now it had been easy to ignore; it had been easy to deny. I had kicked it under the bed with all my half-read books. I thought I'd get back to it and deal with it later. But it got back to me first. RA was truly forcing itself into my life. No longer could I convince myself that the disease didn't exist. How much longer could I pretend that I was healthy like my friends? I started to feel the burden of my secret.

Though Geoff tried to support me through these attacks—which I called 'flares'—as a young, healthy man, my condition was beyond his comprehension. He did, however, learn to use my RA as a way to gain greater control over me. I believed him when he said that no-one, except him, would ever love me because of my illness. I didn't know it then, but I'd carry this feeling with me for many years to come.

There were some things, however, that I did know—and that knowledge was grim. I wasn't going to be the carefree, blonde, Aussie girl who lived happily ever after with her sports star boyfriend; there was never to be another family Christmas at our Black Rock home and, for my entire life, I wouldn't be free of this devil inside.

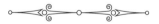

I may not have had the strength to break up with Geoff if it weren't for another break I had to make: I quit Qantas. I loved this great

Australian airline, but my body couldn't take it and my heart wasn't in it. I'd always loved children and I began applying to schools where I could pursue a teaching degree. I was overjoyed and full of enthusiasm when I was accepted for teacher training at Melbourne's Christ College.

I told Geoff we were through, I'd had enough. It turned out he hadn't.

The first week of my new career training—orientation week—ended with an evening of bar-hopping with new university friends. I was late coming home to Black Rock that balmy Friday night in February, my head still spinning with jukebox tunes from the Saint Kilda nightclub Bojangles.

Three years on, this club would become infamous for the carpark killing of 'Sammy the Turk' by Melbourne underground figure Chopper Read. Fancy going there, I thought later, acknowledging that my decision to kick on and party at this seedy bar was not a smart one. It was, however, a sad reflection of my defiant state of mind and of the lack of responsibility I felt towards myself. I couldn't be told anything by anyone.

As I trudged up the dark driveway to the front door of my home, I heard a voice call my name and instantly froze.

'I saw that piece of shit Andrew drop you off,' Geoff said.

The streetlight etched his figure in the black shadows of trees. Where was his car?

'Go home, Geoff,' I said. 'We're not together anymore.'

'You think you're so good don't you? You think you're gonna be the next Miss Australia don't ya? Mum and Dad have chucked me out and I think I'm off Saint Kilda's list because you've f**ked up my pre-season.'

I didn't reply, but turned my back on him and continued walking towards the front door. I never made it.

'Don't you walk away from me,' he bellowed.

In a few quick strides Geoff caught up and shoved me to the ground. The last thing I saw was his scuffed black boot coming in fast—I'd been tackled by a footballer's strongest weapon. My wrists were too swollen to break the fall. I hit the ground with a thud, smashing my head on the concrete.

Kick, kick, kick, kick…Old Mrs Walsh, who lived across the road, counted 16 kicks to my head.

After kicking me into oblivion, Geoff immediately began to protest his innocence. I could hear him as I floated in and out of consciousness.

'Some guys from down the road…at, at the party…they attacked you, then me. Are, are you okay? What do you want to do?'

I was utterly confused. My face felt numb and there was blood on my hands. Geoff scooped me off the footpath, helped me to my feet, put me in the car and began to drive me to a friend's house. As we headed off, my brother, Steve, shot past after his night shift at the yacht club. Geoff tooted the horn and waved as if nothing had happened.

Five minutes later, my friends opened their door to see me with a bloodied nose, swollen eyes and a contorted face covered with abrasions. They knew Geoff's temper. They knew it had to be him. His story didn't fly with them but, in my confusion, I didn't know what to believe.

'Call Steve. Call the police.'

Chapter 3
Reason to Believe

Suddenly, I was part of the battered woman cliché. I played the role beautifully and chose to go on being with my abuser. That was a disaster, but there was worse to come.

The hours after the attack are still a blur in my mind. I was aware I was questioned by the police and that I was taken to hospital. It was 1.30 a.m. Later I received a copy of the letter sent to the police by the ear, nose and throat surgeon, John Castello, who attended me in hospital. Addressed to Constable Hughes, it said, inter alia:

> *On examination of Karen Ager, bruising was noted about the face. Bruising was noted specifically about the left eye and orbit. There were grazes over the bridge of the nose…examination of the mouth showed evidence of a malocclusion, that is the teeth were not able to be placed together in a normal fashion…X-rays showed a fracture of the lower right jaw in two places… It is my opinion that the injuries she suffered were consistent with being assaulted by blows to the face.*

I spent time in the hospital's intensive care unit after the doctors wired my jaws shut, but have little memory of it; I was void of emotion. My spirit and teenage innocence had been bashed out of me and I knew it. RA was taking my body and the assault had taken my heart. The girl who arrived home was a mere shadow of the girl who had so happily gone off to party the previous Friday night. I had black eyes, a bruised and bloated face and a mouth I couldn't open. I couldn't eat, sleep or speak. Nor, unbelievably, could I be reasoned with. Alone amongst family and friends, I clung to the fiction of assault by anonymous partygoers and parroted Geoff's alibi.

However, I couldn't fool my fellow students at Christ College. I was *the girl who'd been bashed by her boyfriend.*

As an abused female, I was no rarity in our macho culture where roughly one in five young women between the ages of 18 and 24 are a victim of domestic violence. In the US the statistics are worse—in the States a woman is battered every nine seconds.

I learned pretty quickly that there's no solidarity in these sad statistics; all but one of my new friends avoided me. Vicky and I must have looked an odd couple walking the halls and hanging out between classes—a short, bubbly brunette in baggy men's sweaters and a willowy blonde with a pair of silver pliers on a chain around her neck.

Mum, who had once again flown home to Melbourne to be by my side, had shown Vicky how to loosen the wires in my mouth in case I choked on food. She insisted I wear the pliers until my jaw healed. I looked ridiculous with these as a fashion accessory, but Vicky made me laugh—albeit through clenched teeth—as she acted out all the scenarios which required automatic jaw opening.

Mum stayed on at the Black Rock house until I was 'wire free'. It seemed as if all she had done since she left was 'come home'. She pureed roast dinners and made me energy drinks. The family put all their differences aside and pulled together after the assault and it felt good to me. I felt closer to Mum than I had in years. In a strange twist, the bashing had helped breach the gap between us. She had shown me that near or far, married or separated, she was there when I needed her. I began to feel less abandoned.

Geoff was charged with two counts of assault—assault causing actual bodily harm and assault causing grievous bodily harm—and was facing a term in jail. When I arrived at the Court House in Sandringham I had decided to save Geoff from a jail term by dropping the most serious charge—assault causing grievous bodily harm.

Mum understood, but Steve and Dad were horrified. I think Mum knew that my disease had made me fragile and that I had depended on Geoff for emotional support. As a result of being manipulated by Geoff I had become isolated from my family and the feeling of being utterly alone compounded my vulnerability.

Though I didn't understand the side effects of my disease, RA had already mentally disabled me and I'd become trapped in my relationship with Geoff because of my disability. RA had prolonged my abuse. It had delayed my decision to leave him. Though I saved him from a jail sentence, Geoff's final punishment underlined the seriousness with which the courts viewed his actions. He was given a criminal conviction, a 12-month probation order to stay away from me and an order to stay out of the state of Victoria for three years.

The stress of this mess precipitated a full-scale battle with my disease. It picked up speed to advance fearlessly in its quest to overcome me. The cortisone injections in my shoulders and knees were powerful weapons in this war, but the relief was short and it was never very long before the next army of attackers marched towards the front-line.

The massive doses of oral cortisone did nothing to stop the degeneration of my joints. Swallowing these tablets was like wearing a mask. The medication masked the pain but not the deformity. Conventional drugs were no longer controlling my illness at all. I was living with constant uncertainty about my future.

I did believe that Geoff had loved me despite all of my problems and I missed his support. As time passed and the disease progressed, I began to lose all hope of meeting anyone who would love me and take on the burden of my chronic illness. I was a lost soul. Intimacy equalled pain and I'd had enough of that

Studying, however, provided a precious measure of happiness. I tried not to care about my reputation as the girl who was assaulted. In my first year of teacher training I began practice teaching rounds. What a thrill! The children were curious and engaging and I felt a surge of pride each time I stood before them, leading them through their lessons, answering questions and showing them how to use reference materials to find answers on their own.

In teaching I had found the career for which I yearned. Innately I understood that to make a difference I had to find a way of connecting with each child I taught. If Henry liked planes, then I'd tell him about the aviation careers of my father and my brother. The next day, there would be Henry, bolting into class to present me with a carefully coloured picture of a jumbo jet. I understood that making connections with each child would help them feel that I cared—and spur them on to learn. It was one of the secrets of being a good teacher and it came to me naturally.

One of the classroom teachers I did my 'prac' with used to jog his Year 5 class around the block before lessons began.

'They'll settle down more quickly if they've burnt off their morning energy,' he said.

I couldn't run, but I didn't want to tell the teacher, Mr Campaciaili, that. Such an admission could have influenced his report on me and caused me to fail that teaching round. My solution to the problem was to hang back with the overweight kids and the uncoordinated ones—pretending that I was keeping tabs on the tail-enders. As we attempted to pound the neighbourhood pavement I don't doubt that their thoughts were just like mine.

Puffing along they would gasp: 'I can't keep up. I'll never finish. I hope Mr C's not looking. I'm not as good as everyone else.'

These children had no idea how much I identified with them. They were comforted by my presence at the back of the line as we half-walked and half-skipped together—and I was so relieved that, in the practice-teaching context, my RA continued to be my secret.

Teaching forced me to search for answers to the 'why me' question I'd been asking myself for years about my disease. These kids saw my inability to run and I saw their inadequacies without passing judgement. For those brief moments, I wasn't a teacher; I was a friend who understood.

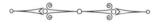

After graduating, in January 1987 I went to work as a kindergarten teacher at St Kevin's Primary School in Ormond, a short drive from the Melbourne suburb of Sandringham. I lived in a two-bedroom house Mum bought after the sale of our family home at Black Rock.

My parents had divorced and Dad was back on the dating scene. That was weird. He continued to be like a nutty professor—void of common sense but always great fun to be with. I went to visit him one day and scribbled down the phone number of a girlfriend and accidentally left it on his bedside table. After I left, he saw the number—written on the back of one of his business cards—and figured that it was the number of a woman he'd recently met. He rang the number.

'Hi, Deborah. You probably don't remember me, but my name's Max Ager we met on an overnight and I was wondering if you'd like to go out on a date?'

'An overnight? What's that? Look, I don't know a Max Ager but I do go to teachers' college with Karen Ager.'

The whole episode was 'very Max'.

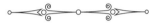

My brother was now a pilot with Qantas and I was a 23-year-old teacher with a new car, a nice 'pad' and an inferiority complex the size of Ayers Rock—or Uluru as the massive monolith in the middle of Australia is now called.

Though I could spot the anxieties of my students at a glance, I couldn't get a handle on my own. After my assault more than three years earlier, I was too spooked to date. Geoff, who had lived in Perth since he was banished from Victoria by the court, had served his time and was back in Melbourne for the football season. He phoned me every day.

I was lonely and listened to him as he told me how much he missed me. He claimed our love was true and promised to love me even though I was sick.

I wish I'd known then that women with disabilities experience the highest rate of personal violence against them. If one in five young women are assaulted—according to those who provide the statistics—then one in every two or three with disabilities can expect abuse. When the football season ended Geoff went back to Perth, begging me to come live with him. As soon as the school year ended, I did—against the loudly voiced advice and wishes of all the members of my family.

The irony of moving to be with Geoff, in the city to which he had fled after the court order to leave me alone, was lost on me. Mum wasn't even living there anymore. The relationship for which she had held such high hopes following the separation from my father had proved a disappointment and she'd moved to the southern suburbs of Sydney to be closer to her brothers and sister.

Geoff met me at the airport with his arms full of cream-coloured roses and off we went in yet another Holden—this one a sleek sedan that came with his new job as a salesman.

As soon as I had settled in with Geoff I dropped my curriculum vitae (CV) off to the headmasters of local schools. Within a very short time I had a full schedule of substitute teaching in a working-class neighbourhood. The work was varied, demanding and challenging, but I loved it—along with the children of battlers that I taught. Professional fulfillment, however, couldn't change the fact that, by moving to Perth and back into Geoff's arms and life, I had made a huge blunder.

It didn't take him long to fall into his old patterns of bullying me. I began to understand that my ill-judged partnership choice was symptomatic of my disease. I also became acutely aware that my ability to protect myself had become very limited. I'd distanced myself from Mum and detached from Steve and Dad, who were still disappointed about my decision to be with Geoff. I began to grasp that by positioning myself away from my family in the most isolated city in the world, I'd given Geoff all the control and power over me that he could ever want. I was powerless and this feeling was intensified by the presence of my disease. I felt trapped. I was desperately looking for a way out when fate played a role and rescued me from my predicament.

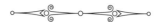

A group of girlfriends had taken off for an overseas holiday and invited me to join them. It was the sort of thing that many Aussies do in their 20s—after they have their career qualifications and before they settle down to permanent employment. When I accepted their invitation, little did I know the separation from Geoff would be final. If this had entered my head I know I would have succumbed to all the vulnerabilities that I felt and these insecurities would have overruled any decision to leave. It was a lucky escape.

My girlfriends were on a grand tour of Europe in a Volkswagen Kombi van and I caught up with them in Rome. Lisa, my mischievous childhood companion, was my caretaker. Friends since our mothers gave birth to us two days apart, Lisa and I were complete opposites. She was brunette, I was blonde. She was short, I was tall. She was the troublemaker and the one in control. I was the goody-goody-two-shoes and the follower.

And she was so naughty! I revelled in her antics even though the joke was often on me.

'C'mon, Kaz,' Lisa would say when we were kids.

'Give me your lollies and I'll save them for you...I really will.'

I knew she was the Candy Queen but I'd believe her promises—only to find myself misled and locked in a cupboard while she munched away on my chocolate freckles, golden bananas and jelly beans. Sometimes she'd swim up behind me, loosen my bikini bra ties and whisk it away, leaving me topless to tread water amongst the snorkellers at Black Rock beach.

Lisa was like a sister to me and even though we had our moments I knew that she'd always be there for me—to the end. I was never really sure why she picked me to be one of her European travel companions because, to have me there meant lifting and lugging my suitcases—as well as her own—while I shuffled along behind.

The other girls were Lisa's friends from Sydney who had also become my friends over the years. Margo was short with thick, blonde hair. She was super-sensitive but could be hilariously funny. Sometimes she seemed closer to me than to Lisa. The other two girls could only be described as 'the glamourpusses'. Super-looking and sexy, they oozed sensuality, with Elle Macpherson bodies, sun-kissed skin and the sporty appeal of the all-Australian woman. They were everything Margo, Lisa and I were not.

As soon as my aircraft landed in Italy my joints protested. From Rome we went on a bouncy drive south to the port of Brindisi and from there on to a ferry to the Greek island of Paros.

Grinding hours of immobility in plane, car and boat—two days of non-stop travel since my mumbled goodbye to Geoff—caused a massive flare-up. I countered with double doses of my prescriptions, further medicating myself with beer, wine, ouzo and whatever else was being poured. I was determined to have a good time, to keep up with the other girls, whatever the cost.

Our first night in Paros ended when the Aussie fivesome plus two cute Americans sneaked keys past a hotel's reception desk and helped ourselves to accommodations. Bleary and still half-blotto in the morning, we decided to slip from our rooms and scale the property's high stucco wall—a getaway I couldn't come close to accomplishing. After the others went up and over the whitewashed wall, I limped to the front desk, handed our keys to a dumbstruck clerk and rushed as fast as my wonky legs could carry me to the idling van.

As stupid and selfish as these antics were, they felt liberating. We partied all night, every night. Massive doses of cortisone elevated me to feeling 'normal', like my friends.

'Thank God for the cortisone,' Lisa and I would shout as we threw back another shot of tequila, both happy that I wasn't missing—in the least—the man who had bashed me.

But I didn't go unpunished. In the weeks ahead, the compound insults I inflicted on my body took their toll. My ride on a Santorini donkey down the side of a steep cliff almost ended in disaster. I couldn't hold on to the donkey's reins because of my swollen fingers and inflamed and sore wrists. Falling sideways, saddle and all, I couldn't pull myself back up. A Greek 'donkey walker' with no knowledge of the English language and a donkey happily trotting down the cliff were in control.

'Could you please stop?' I asked.

There was no response.

'STOP.'

Still there was no response.

'Stop the f***ing donkey.' My frantic yell carried a note of desperation.

Suddenly the Greek man understood English. I was both crying and laughing.

I saw the comedy in this absurd situation—but it was an acute reminder of my own frailties and of how I couldn't do the things that my friends were able to do. As much as I didn't want to believe it, I was beginning to understand that I just wasn't like them. The end of the party was looming.

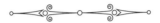

In May I said a sad farewell to my friends and left for Holland to spend time with Steve and Mum in her home country.

From the moment we were reunited I felt Mum was examining me closely. I hobbled through a tour of her birth city, Groningen, but when we moved on to Paris I was bedridden with pain. Her heart broke as, together with Steve and Lisa's Dad, Jack, she climbed the steps of the Notre Dame Cathedral while I waited behind—a cripple.

After that numbing experience, Mum dropped her bombshell.

I wouldn't be rejoining my girlfriends in the south of Portugal as planned, she said. Instead, I was headed for an arthritis clinic in England where a retired nurse named Margaret Hills would rid me of my illness.

Mum had been researching RA and had read Margaret's book *Curing Arthritis the Drug Free Way*. Having been aware of my deterioration, she was at the point of losing all hope and, in a move born of despair, persuaded herself that the all-natural methods advocated in the book would be my salvation. It was the last resort of a mother to save her daughter.

Knowing I would protest, Mum flew to the other side of the world to 'ambush' me after our holiday in Holland with Steve. Our time in Paris reassured her she was doing the right thing. Traditional medications were not controlling my disease and I was in trouble. She knew it and, deep down, so did I. Apart from the pain of seeing her daughter's body deform in front of her eyes, I think Mum feared she would have a sickly daughter to look after for the rest of her life.

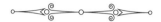

There was no scientific evidence to prove that Margaret Hills' alternative therapies would work for arthritis as aggressive as mine. But here we were on our way to Coventry and to the clinic. Testimonials and a personal reply from Margaret Hills to a letter Mum had written were enough. But, that was typical of my 'gung-ho' Mum: *I have to fix it and I have to do it now.*

It turned out that Mum was not alone in her thinking. It is estimated that 90 per cent of all people with arthritis will turn to alternative medicine at some point. If there was a chance I'd be cured there was no stopping Mum.

I was too weak to fight. I shuffled from our hotel in the heart of Paris to the closest Metro subway station. Our first destination was Charles de Gaulle airport. We waved goodbye to Jack as the metro whisked us away. He was bound for The Algarve, Portugal, to see Lisa, but his face told me that he was worried for our family.

Walking through Customs at London's Heathrow airport, I couldn't believe I was in England. I had never been there before nor did I ever have the desire to visit. Listening to the accents around me I felt the usual unfounded disdain that Aussies feel towards the 'Poms'.

'I don't like the drool, don't like the place and I don't want to be here,' I ranted.

I resented Mum for doing this. I deeply begrudged the way she'd sprung the idea on me. I was angry at her for making me go to England. I already felt as if I had no control in my life. This decision was made for me and I was very annoyed about it. What was most upsetting was that I wouldn't be meeting up with the girls in Portugal for another few weeks of carefree bar-hopping. There was no way I'd be well enough or finished with the all-natural treatment in time to join them.

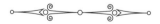

Back in Australia, Dad was in denial about my disease. He hadn't seen me for some months. He did not know how sick I was, nor could he see how RA had physically deformed me. The idea of having an invalid daughter was just not in his realm of thinking. I was his 'princess'.

When Dad was told of my condition, the resultant stress prompted a reaction—the classic fight or flight response. He chose the latter. Was he abandoning me? I didn't allow myself to think that—not of my Dad. The side effect of his absence was that Mum was forced to deal with the multiple problems of having a crippled daughter on her own, while fumbling around England without much money. Steve took on a fatherly role and worried about leaving us so far from home.

'I am not going until I've found somewhere in Coventry for you to live,' Steve promised. The city of Coventry, about an hour and a half north-west of London, was dull and morbid-looking. Black clouds hung overhead and a strange ambience pervaded the atmosphere. It seemed to engulf me. I didn't know why it felt like that until I learned about the loss of life in that region during World War II.

Coventry was one of the most heavily bombed cities in England and still bore many of the scars of war. The city was a prime target because of its many munitions factories. Roofs were painted black to create a sea of darkness, no lights were allowed at night and thick curtains attempted to shut out the world. Coventry Cathedral was completely destroyed in 1940 during a blitz in this industrial city which killed 554 and injured hundreds of others. Today a blackened and burnt timber cross rests on the altar. The words *Father Forgive* are emblazoned behind it.

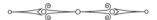

Steve set out with Mum to find lodgings for us. It was not easy in Coventry. A poor currency exchange rate meant we couldn't afford much. Shared accommodation appeared to be our only option. For a while it looked like Mum and I would be living in a bed-sitter with two elderly men who sat at home all day and drank. Boozing veterans perched in front of the television day and night would certainly not help my recovery.

Then a miracle happened.

Our angel was an elderly lady called Ann. She was short and stocky and could have been cast in a film as a 'tea lady'. Her accent was heavy in the style of what the locals called 'West country farmer's'. In Coventry the word *that* is pronounced *thut* and *them* is said as *thum*. All very strange to the ears of an Aussie.

Ann had heard about my story at the Margaret Hills Clinic. When she met Mum she saw the desperation in her eyes. She opened her heart to us and for £38 a week she gave us her home while she moved in with one of her adult children. Mum and I had somewhere to live while I was in treatment.

I took this generosity as a sign that this was where I was meant to be for now. Mum and I moved into Ann's small, one-bedroom unit in Green Lane, Coventry. Sharing a bed was a small price to pay.

We said goodbye to Steve on another grey morning in the carpark of a city bus depot in Coventry. In this moment I understood how deep my brother's love for me was and how he too had been hurt by my disease. We were all afflicted. RA had damaged us all. Holding back tears, Mum and I waved goodbye as Steve's Heathrow-bound bus accelerated away.

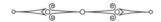

The Margaret Hills Clinic was in a white clapboard house. Mrs Hills, a matronly former nurse—in support stockings and flat shoes—sat me down and outlined a plan to wean me from all my medications and purge my body of toxins. She had cured her own RA, she said and many others as well.

I went to the clinic every day for almost two months. The new regime began with me drinking apple cider vinegar and taking molasses three times per day, together with vitamin C, omega-3, calcium and cod liver oil pills—all meticulously dispensed in Ziploc bags. This was known as the 'Margaret Hills Formula'. The cider vinegar, though not really pleasant, was acceptable, but the molasses tasted foul. I was proud of myself because in less than a week I had cut my prescribed medications by half. What I didn't understand was that this goal was a dangerous one. Anyone who has been on oral cortisone—prednisone—should know that you have to wean yourself off the tablets, slowly reducing the dosage by a few milligrams a day. Stopping 'cold turkey' could send me into a downward spiral. In my journal I recorded my thoughts over those dismal days in 1988:

28 May: Today I thought about the drugs I am on—gold, feldene and cortisone—and I've decided the sooner I stop them, the more chance I have of getting my body back to normal and of letting this new treatment work. Yep, I'm going off all drugs as soon as I can. I am going to attack this damn disease head on. I can't be selfish and say I am doing it for me. No, I'll do it for Mum and Steve because they want so much for me to be well. I WILL make this work and I WILL get better.

30 May: I have had two really bad days. There are the usual pains—fingers, wrists, shoulders, feet etc.—but I also have dreadful pain in my muscles from my knees to my hips. I am unable to get off the couch, sit on the toilet or walk. Please God help me to get better. Please make this work.

31 May—Mum's birthday: Happy birthday, Mum! I WILL get better and give her the best birthday present she would ever want. She WILL have a healthy daughter! So I am following Margaret Hills' diet religiously and swallowing all the stuff she prescribes a few times a day to balance my acidity levels. I am lucky that Mum has the patience to shuffle with me, cook and clean and rub me when I am sore. I have terrible pain under my right boob on my chest. She rubbed me, but I'm frustrated at not being able to roll over or move myself on the bed. I can't lie on either side. We both cried. I can't imagine Mum's pain when she sees me like this.

1 June: We went to the clinic today. Mrs Hills was happy with my progress because I am now able to wash my own face and lift a plate with one hand. When I see her I feel a sense of calm. I am now more determined than ever to get over this. Especially, when I am with this amazing woman and I know how much she has suffered and what courage she has. I pray that I will find the same bravery. Mum has had to find a job to pay the rent—she has been working for 90 pounds a week doing some accounting. She comes home really tired. My days are long without her.

4 June: It is my birthday and how lonely I feel. I am improving but there's still a lot of pain. My jaw is sore so I can't eat or open my mouth properly to clean my teeth. My hips, my knees, my toes all ache. I can't brush my hair, carry a cup or cut up my dinner. My wrists are so sore that I can't pull up my own undies.

6 June: I had a consultation with Mrs Hills. She is happy that I have less pain today in some of my joints. She says my progress is good. I always leave the clinic with renewed hope and determination. I aim to be as courageous as Mrs Hills and as caring as Mum. I feel I can do this. I can beat this thing.

11 June: Again I am being told my progress is good, but to be honest I don't feel it or see it. I have sore feet and sore hands. I am sore everywhere! I am also feeling really isolated as I haven't had any letters from home. I'm watching *Neighbours* on television everyday just to feel connected to Australia.

19 June: I went to Stratford-Upon-Avon, the home of Shakespeare, with Mum and her work friends. It was good to get out, but I'd worked myself up so much about whether I would be capable of walking around that I ruined it for myself. I didn't know these people and felt embarrassed. I put myself under a lot of pressure to appear to walk normally.

20 June: I am so tired after being out yesterday. All I want to do is sleep. But the good news is Mrs Hills told me that Mum and I can make plans to leave the clinic early in July. My biggest progress is that I'm walking around without being on medication. She says I'll keep improving and I can finish my recuperation at home in Australia.

21 June: I'm all right but I'm walking on the outside of my feet because of the pain. My legs are sore and when Mum rubs me she says she feels ridges under the surface of the skin. God my body is riddled with RA. I am very weak right now and I am not feeling at all confident about the almighty trip home to Oz. I feel scared about the flight.

By the time I was ready to fly home my ankles and knees were swollen to twice their normal size, the stiffness in my elbows prevented me from straightening my arms and my right shoulder jutted forward—the bones had reconfigured into a bulbous new shape. My right hip was so painful I kept my arm down to shield it, terrified a bump would send a bolt of pain down my leg that would bring me to my aching knees. Fewer than a hundred pounds hung on my crooked six-foot frame. I convinced myself that this was all just part of the healing process.

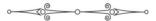

Mum turned 50 while we were in Coventry. I am guessing it was the saddest birthday that she ever had. I felt distressed that her life was on hold because of me. I felt even sadder that she had been the one who had copped the brunt of my bad feelings. The one I'd sought to blame for my disease. But all she wanted was a healthy daughter. I continued to convince myself as I swallowed an assortment of brews and concoctions that I would be better soon.

I turned 24 while at the Coventry clinic and had been weaned from all medication—thoroughly 'detoxed' in the Hills' vernacular. I flew home with Mum and moved into her apartment in the Sydney suburb of Sans Souci. We both still had hope. Hope that I'd soon be well.

Hope! Is it always the last thing to go?

Chapter 4
Horror Movie

Marooned in a fourth-floor walk-up apartment, unable to dress or wash myself—or even use the bathroom alone—I sank into an immobile stupor under the government-subsidised care of my mum.

The suburb, south of Sydney, was Sans Souci which is French for *without worries* or *carefree*. I doubt the irony was lost on anyone who knew me when I returned to Australia on 4 July 1988. I was carried up to Mum's condo like a bundle of laundry by Lisa's Dad, Jack, who gently placed me on the narrow bed that had once worn my lime-green, daisy duvet back in Black Rock.

Crippled and withered as a crone, helpless as a newborn, I spent restless nights in my childhood bed. My torpid days dragged on the couch watching the blue rhythms of Botany Bay through a picture window. Books were too heavy for my hands. TV was a bore. My world was unchanging and I was stuck in the midst of its cycle of tedious repetition.

When my RA was flaring my wrists were my enemy. I needed Mum for everything. She'd dress me because raising my arms above my head was impossible. I'd sit on the bed like a four-year-old while she held my clothes, placed the shirt over my head and then carefully threaded each arm through the sleeves. I needed Mum to lift the tea cup to my mouth and, watching her cut my food into manageable pieces, I felt useless. Next, I would try to feed myself, my left arm at an awkward angle because of my swollen elbow. Chewing was tough—another simple task which was now too hard because of RA in my jaw. Brushing my teeth with palpable awkwardness was a sight

I preferred not to view in the mirror on the wall.

I was off all my 'meds' as dictated by the Margaret Hills' RA remedy, but I was beginning to wonder what the point of it all was if I couldn't do anything for myself—not even walk. Freeing me of my medication had been my goal and, even though I had my doubts, I was still determined to follow the drug-frees cure as formulated by the British former nurse. I didn't want doctors involved because I knew they would be condemnatory. I had set out to rid myself of the medication and the toxins in my body at the Margaret Hills Clinic and no-one was going to take this goal away from me—even if I couldn't walk. I wanted to defy the odds.

The balls of my feet hurt like I was walking on pebbled ground. My ankles were swollen like watermelons and my knees had become balloons filled with fluid. Every step I took hurt like hell. The pain was unimaginable. I figured out that somehow there was less soreness if I put my heel on the ground first and rolled the rest of my foot down. This way I could step 'off my joints'. When I moved from room to room in the apartment I shuffled with the gait of a Neanderthal. One morning, while hobbling to the bathroom, I became conscious of the fact that walking, perhaps the most basic human activity, had become an isolating experience. It was isolating because every step was painful and because it caused people to stare at me. I felt self-conscious, embarrassed and maybe even ashamed about the way I shuffled along. Balancing on my two feet to stand even semi-upright or to sit down was hard too. Perhaps bystanders stared because they thought I'd had too much to drink—or perhaps just because they felt sorry for me. I did not know, but I chose not to meet the eyes of passersby. Instead, I looked down at the ground. It was less confrontational—but it became a habit which was hard to break. With each solitary step I began to feel deep down that I was in this on my own.

I was also self-conscious about my physical appearance. My body was skin and bone, pin-thin and could hardly bear its own weight. My joints had a mind of their own and were bullying me. My right hip buckled beneath me and I no longer trusted it. My bloated elbows bossed my arms, not allowing them to straighten out. It was like there was an army within pushing my shoulder forward until it, too, warped and took on a new form. My once-attractive figure was crooked and bent. I was no longer symmetrical. The illness was deforming my body right before my eyes. There was nothing I could do to stop the distortion, or to stop my entire frame from collapsing beneath me.

RA was sentencing me to a lifetime of pain and disability. It was relentless. Everything seemed hopeless. I knew my disease was now defining me and I began to believe that the skeletal person who stared back at me from the mirror was the 'new me' and that this struggle was my destiny. I was angry that Margaret Hills' formula had not worked for me as it had for others. I was angry at Mum for taking me to Coventry. I was angry at my body, which refused to cooperate with my mind. I was angry at Dad for not being around and I was angry that Steve had the perfect life. I was just angry! The sight of my skinny, misshapen body in the mirror repulsed me and fed my anger. I felt ugly.

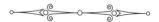

RA was now causing distress in every dimension of my life—my relationships, my work (or lack of it), my spirituality, my recreational time and my mind. It consumed me. I couldn't allow myself to disappear into girlish dreams about boyfriends, weddings and children. Instead my mind was filled with fear about what lay ahead. This fear was beginning to twist my mind as the disease had mangled my body. I became tormented by questions which haunted me day and night, night and day. Who would love me enough to take on this responsibility? Would I ever be able to return to work and teach again? Would my anger ever go away? Why would God do this to me? Would I be able to go out and party with my friends ever again, or would I just lie in my bed, night after night, listening to the footsteps of women in high heels, giggling as they shimmied down the street, on their way to a theatre, a restaurant or a night-club? Would I love again and would I ever have a child? It felt as if my life was on hold with no glimmer of hope.

My fears were all wrapped up with my low self-esteem and my neediness. I didn't know how to break out of this crazy emotional pattern I was now in, or how to face my fears head on. So I chose not to face any of these things at all. If Mum had the same fears she never talked about them with me. However, I knew she must have shared my thoughts.

Sometimes I'd hear her in the night, still awake at 3 a.m. She'd cough a few times, take a sip of water and roll over, trying to fall asleep again. We were the stars in this horror movie and the reel kept on turning. There was no happy ending in sight.

I knew I was wearing Mum down. My RA was wrecking her life as well as mine. We both needed some relief. Mum went back to work part-time and I retreated back to bed. Work provided a bit of an escape for her—and we needed the money. The sickness benefit I received from the Australian Government wasn't enough to pay the bills—even when combined with the cheque Mum received for her duties as my carer.

When Mum went to work the days became almost endless for me, even though she was only working three or four hours at a time. Before she left in the morning she would prop me up on her salmon leather couch in front of the television. She filled a side table with Vegemite sandwiches and a large plastic sports bottle of juice that I drank through a straw, leaning over to sip because my wrists were too weak to hold the bottle. When she returned she helped me to the bathroom and tended me as I went to the toilet. In some horrid way I felt like Mum deserved to have her motherly responsibilities return to her as a kind of penance for having deserted us—for having left home.

I didn't miss Dad much, nor did it bother me anymore that he wasn't around. I knew he couldn't handle his beautiful daughter being sick, so I excused him. The sight of my thin frame would have sent him into a frenzy, so, in my mind, I shut him out and he escaped blame. In hindsight it was all too easy. I didn't even blame Dad for not accepting the responsibility of a sick daughter or for being unavailable. I enabled him to live in denial without blame, while Mum kept dutifully feeding me, dressing me and wiping me clean after visits to the bathroom. Years would pass before I showed her any morsel of gratitude or absolved her of her penance and told her how wonderful she was to me during this time.

Later I would understand how much the fear of abandonment was a thread that was intricately woven into many pivotal points in my life. Mum was disappointed again by Dad and his absence, but, for me, a phone call once in a while was enough. I tried not to shoulder the disillusionment that Mum felt towards my father.

The view of Botany Bay, as beautiful as it was, did little other than frustrate me. Lisa and Margo were now in New York and I tried to imagine what we'd be doing if I were with them.

Daydreaming, I imagined myself walking in Times Square on the way to a Broadway show. I envisaged what it would be like to have conversations with New Yorkers and whether or not I'd understand the rolling twang of their accents. In my mind's eye I was dining with my girlfriends in a swanky New York restaurant. I told myself that I was pain-free. My mind allowed me to forget my world and, just for a moment, I escaped to the Big Apple to be with them.

My daydream was interrupted by the ringing of the phone.

The high-pitched, insistent sound forced me back into my harsh reality. It was a reality that I didn't want to face. I tried to get off the couch to answer the call but my hips, knees, ankles, feet and wrists—all my joints—were frozen. I could hardly move. I couldn't lift my dead weight off the couch, it was too low and I didn't have the strength in my arms to push myself up. The ringing persisted. Somehow I rolled myself off the couch and began to slide along the floor to the kitchen, pushing myself along with the sides of my feet and my elbows because my wrists were too swollen to move. I was motivated to keep moving by the continuing ringing. Finally I got to the kitchen and, pulling myself up by hanging on to the legs of the table, I was high enough to reach the telephone. At that moment the ringing stopped. There I was half on the floor, kneeling awkwardly and crookedly on my knees, unable to stand upright.

I faced the undeniable fact that I could not even answer the telephone by myself. I felt utterly defeated. I rolled my body carefully from the kneeling position to the foetal position and lay crying on the kitchen floor, unable to move. The hours went by and tears streamed down my cheeks on to my chest. I soothed myself by rocking back and forth.

Eventually Mum came home from work. She arrived to find me still crying on the floor, enmeshed in my own pain. The task of getting me back to the couch, for the instant, seemed impossible, so she lay on the kitchen floor too, beside me on the cold tiles. We cried as we clung together. In that moment I understood that she was as desperate as I. The year of Australia's much-celebrated bicentennial, 1988, was proving to be the longest year of my life.

20 August: Yesterday I began to lose faith. Today I am telling myself I can't give up. Mum has booked me into a course called *Mind Powers*. It's probably because of our 'kitchen floor moment'. The course is not really me, but I have agreed to start next Tuesday. I figure if I can learn some strategies to keep myself motivated and to keep believing that I will get better, it could help. I do want to be healthy, I do want to work and to marry one day and to have kids.

Steve's new girlfriend, Trudy, is nice. She's a flight attendant and a dead ringer for Olivia Newton John. It's my family history repeating itself; pilot meets flight attendant. For some reason I believe he'll marry her. Selfishly, I already feel a sense of loss. He is not around as much. But being the amazing brother that he is, he's already read my mind. Unsolicited he told me that no one can replace his sister. 'I've given you all I can as a brother, this is an aspect of me I can't give you, but I'll always be there as your brother.' He said in a phone call. I feel happy for Steve that he's met someone nice. I know I should look at it as a gain rather than a loss; after all I'll gain Trudy as a sister—albeit 'in-law'.

4 September: I'm sitting out on the verandah like an old woman with a rug over my knees and a pillow behind me. It's a pathetic sight. The last month has been awful—possibly the worst in my life. My right hip now collapses beneath me when I try to put weight on it. The pain just hasn't let up. I tried to do the self-help course but it was too painful to get there. Last week I was extremely depressed.

I lost all my will to fight this battle; I couldn't be bothered getting out of bed. For five days I shut myself away from Mum and the rest of the world. All day every day, the pain took over completely. I feel I have no will to beat this anymore. My problems now are many: left foot, right swollen knee, sore right hip, tightness in collar bone and jaw. I have swellings that come and go including on the fingers of my left hand, my wrists and shoulders. GODDDDDD, please give me the courage that I need to go on. Without Mum I know I couldn't survive this—she picks me up when I am down and listens patiently when I cry every day. She's my arms and my legs. I was so desperate that I even rang Mrs Hills the other day. Steve's away on a flying trip and I feel much more needy when he's gone. I'm getting so tired of having to contemplate how I'm going to tackle every little movement. I'm sick of missing out on LIFE!!! I'M SICK OF IT!!!!!

28 September: It is four days after the AFL Grand final between Hawthorn and Melbourne. How my life has changed. I didn't have the energy to watch—or for that matter care—about the Super Bowl of the southern hemisphere this year. I've had a pathetic attitude this whole month. I've wallowed in self pity, been in bed all day every day, not eaten, lost weight, thought about putting myself out of my misery and I know I've been terrible to live with. Well it's about time I snapped out of it especially with the encouragement I've had from family and friends. I AM special! I WILL get better and I WILL help others.

2 October: Swellings—wrists, right knee—huge, left foot, right hip. I weigh just fifty-four kilos (129 pounds) and I'm six feet tall. I'm trying harder to keep positive and pray and tell myself I am specially chosen for this because I can handle it, but the last few days have been shocking. Both wrists 'went' on me—I couldn't move them at all. I was totally dependent on Mum again. If I were a horse they would have shot me by now to put me out of my misery. The other day I couldn't make it to the bathroom in time because of my feet. I had to just stand there and wet the floor, like a toddler who had not been potty-trained. How to lose your self-respect in

40 seconds cold. I am trying my hardest not to withdraw, but it's a constant battle and it feels like I can never win. I don't even want to go out of the apartment anymore because of people staring when I walk. They check me out from head to toe and ogle. Then they don't know what to say. The other day, I felt I had achieved so much because I made it down four flights of stairs, one step at a time and then made it to the letter box. I was so proud. Then a man 'on the outside' looked at me and said: 'Do you always walk like that?' I answered, truthfully: 'Yes, I always walk like this.' To a stranger I looked disabled. The strain is beginning to show on Mum again—we are both battling to keep our spirits up. She's been my carer for months now. I fear she's frustrated about having her own life on hold and I am beginning to feel a shift. Steve's the best brother in the world, but I do sometimes feel envious of his career and lifestyle flying around the world in perfect health. Right now it seems easier to withdraw. I'd rather isolate myself than constantly whine. I sometimes feel those around me have everything I've ever dreamed of. God, give me the courage to go on…please God.

Even though I didn't seek, nor want the pity of my family and friends, I knew I was slipping into a cycle of self-pity—and that was dangerous.

8 October: I find solace in my bed because the days are so long and lonely. Today I slept until 1 p.m. and now it's only 2.30 p.m. I want the day to be over. I have had some okay days since I last wrote in my journal, but just when I'm beginning to feel more confident another joint 'goes'. This time it's not one knee but both of my knees. They are so swollen with fluid. I've never seen my left knee so fat and ballooned with fluid. It looks like the skin is about to pop and my leg feels like it weighs a ton. I can't get about at all. I can't get off the loo by myself and am unable to get out of the bath. I am so discouraged and with too much time to think I'm beginning to ask myself whether I am being punished for something. If I knew that there was a certain time limit to this I could cope. Why, I ask myself, would God do this to me? I've been raised to believe in

God, but why is he hurting me? I am beginning to wonder what I
am being punished for. Was it that I didn't go with my mum when
she left home? Mum's great and so is Steve with their never-ending
support and love. I rely on them so much these days that I worry
about losing them and pray that I won't. The Australian cricketer,
Simon O'Donnell, is battling cancer and he is my inspiration right
now. Whenever I get negative thoughts I think of him.

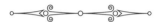

I continued to wage my war against the disease without traditional
medication, still believing that natural remedies would eventually
work for me. Mum, who had researched and guided my way to Mrs
Hills, was not so sure.

She enlisted the help of another matronly nurse, an holistic
something-or-other with yellowed, untended toenails poking out
from her dusty sandals. The woman questioned me and left with a
vial of my blood, phoning later to report that I had food allergies and
should immediately strike from my diet all meat, alcohol, sugar, dairy,
apples, oranges, potatoes and wheat. Her prescribed diet: pineapples
(okay), vegetables (fine) and millet seed (positively curative).

I tried the course of therapy but quit when more weight dropped
from my wasted frame. There wasn't much in life to like at this point.
It was dawning on me that I couldn't go on living like this. Where
was the joy?

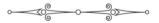

On 26 October 1988 I consulted a rheumatologist. I was increasingly
distressed that, at just 24, my life had become a burden to myself
and to all those around me. In a surprise visit Dad travelled north
from Melbourne to Sydney for the appointment and Mum was by
my side as always. It felt good that Dad was around and trying to
come to grips with the idea that his daughter had a disabling disease.
Again Mum and Dad were uniting for my sake and leaving their
differences behind.

The walls of Dr Reisman's surgery were a sickly shade of custard. Crooked pictures of some pseudo-impressionist's floral art covered gaps on the walls and delivered to my searching eyes no clue about the doctor's personality. His desk was piled with papers, more on the left than right. Perhaps that was a clue. A quick examination and a few X-rays was all it took to determine his first course of action.

'You'll need to have both knees injected with Depomedrol and Xylocaine today.'

I did not question the doctor about the drugs or what side effects I could expect—I was too busy trying to manipulate my body into the treatment room. Mum and Dad remained in the consulting room. I sat psyching myself into getting through this 'multi-injection moment'. Since the age of eight, when I had to be inoculated against smallpox and cholera before a family holiday in Fiji, I had suffered from a fear—almost a phobia—of injections. On that occasion, squirming and hysterical, I had finally been cornered and treated under the desk of the family's general practitioner.

Half naked in my green hospital gown, I thought about that day and felt as vulnerable as that disease-free eight-year-old as I sat on the chair next to the treatment table. Dr Reisman returned to prepare the two syringes as I sat and waited, staring again at the Van Gogh-style flower prints on his walls. I looked around the room trying to distract myself by counting the number of times I could find the word 'sterile'. I was at twelve when the doctor's explanation interrupted me.

'Xylocaine is a local anaesthetic which will ease the pain when I inject the prednisone or Depomedrol, which is a steroid. It will reduce the swelling and bring you relief.'

Even though Mum and Dad were right outside waiting for me I began to panic. It was a solitary moment, etching in my brain the reality of facing my health problems on my own. Ready or not I was being forced to take sole ownership of my disease. I was too sick to have a choice so I braced myself. As the syringe pierced my skin my body became rigid. Attempting to get a grip on my emotions I told myself to think happy thoughts. I chanted 'be strong', be strong,' but it did little to stop the tears from running down my cheeks. It was useless. My sadness had been unchanged with one prick of the needle. I was grieving for my healthy body. I wept, not just because of the pain, but because of the stark reality of my situation. I believed I'd failed in my efforts to conquer the disease without drugs and that by going back to conventional medicine and a RA specialist, I disappointed my family.

Mum came into the treatment room and helped me dress. I felt upset, even ashamed at myself for crying, but when our eyes met I knew she didn't want her daughter to be a hero, she just wanted me to be well. I was beginning to understand that all she wanted was for me to get better.

Hand in hand we returned to the consultation room where Dad was waiting. He was quiet and looked sad. His puppy-dog eyes told me that he knew it was not just time for me to face the facts about my disease, but it was time for him to do that too. He could no longer ignore its onslaught. So we sat and listened to the cocktail of medications that Dr Reisman was prescribing which, hopefully, would lead to me regaining control of my disease.

The doctor had a methodical and brusque way about him as he sat speaking and peering over the top of his black-framed glasses. I knew his goal was to restore some sort of quality to my life—and not to have sympathy for me or my family. I also sensed he felt that I was somewhat responsible (or that my parents had been irresponsible) for creating this demon by going off my 'meds'.

I hobbled out of the doctor's office leaning on Mum with one hand, a wad of prescriptions in the other. Dad lagged behind, not because of our pace, but because he was in shock after learning just how sick his daughter really was.

Those prescriptions were the beginning of a new regimen. They included anti-inflammatories for now; immune suppressants and intravenous steroids in the near future. My 'cocktail' would be taken morning and night, *shaken and not stirred,* forever and a day. I was told to begin immediately to get me back on my feet.

The drive home from Miranda across the Captain Cook Bridge where Botany Bay meets the Georges River was predictably quiet. A few days later a follow-up letter, typed in bold black ink, was sent to my local doctor in Sans Souci. Dr Reisman was precise about my prognosis:

> *Clearly, Miss Ager has severe rheumatoid arthritis. I had a general chat with her and her parents about this. I explained that diet (apart from omega-3 fatty acids) has no part to play in the treatment of arthritis. I advised her to continue with heat and a Faradic stimulator that her father had bought. There are a number of treatment options available to her. I explained that her treatment should be aimed at acute relief and to this aim, I have commenced her on Dolobid 500 mg as a trial therapy. I also mentioned to her that occasionally we use large doses of intravenous steroids as a short term measure and she will consider this. I have also arranged for her to have hydrotherapy at Royal Sydney Hospital.*
> *I aspirated each knee and injected them with Depomedrol and Xyclocaine. I have asked her to return for review in a couple of weeks or earlier if necessary.*

So there it was in black and white. There was no denying our defeat. The disease had won. Its victory signalled by the seizing of every joint in my body. It had claimed them all. It seemed too real now and I felt like our efforts in England were truly in vain. We had failed. All my self-discipline, pain, loneliness, isolation and disappointment—and that of my supportive, ever-loving and self-depriving Mum—seemed worthless. The hard work taken away with some scribbled cursive on a prescription pad. Too easy!

The drugs delivered a restoration of dignity, but I still had a long, long way to go. They masked the pain, while the deformity in my joints surged ahead as if there were a prize at the end of the race.

Three times a week Lisa's Dad, Jack, accompanied Mum and me to the local hospital for hydrotherapy sessions. If not for him, I probably wouldn't have ventured out at all. Jack carried me down the stairs and hauled me back up. Jack was fit but he was fifty-ish and I was a dead weight—a regular sack of potatoes. I should have been wrapped in tissue paper too. If my tender joints were knocked while I was being carried the pain would make me physically ill. A glancing contact with the stair railings would erupt into throbbing pain. I'd soon find myself crying again. Tears and deep breathing were my only self-defence. As I was lifted carefully into Mum's car I'd hold my body stiff. Somehow that helped. Jack would lower me to the ground while Mum steadied me from behind. Then they'd help me get my balance until I was ready to attempt getting into the front passenger seat. Every movement took an eternity. My bottom usually went in first. I would 'plonk' myself on to the lambs-wool covers, feeling a small sense of relief that I'd made it down the stairs and half-way into the car. Next, Mum and Jack would warily lift my right leg up and across. Sometimes my leg wouldn't bend at the knee, it was too swollen. Somehow I would have to elevate my butt off the seat to get my leg in the door. Getting me out of the apartment and into the car would sometimes take an hour or more and was physically exhausting not only for me, but also for Jack and Mum.

When I finally arrived at the hospital I was put straight into a wheelchair. The nurses knew our routine and stood, clad in blue uniforms and soft black shoes, at the main entrance of the hospital. Undressing was easier than dressing. However, if the elastic in my knickers was too tight I would not be able to pull them down. And I always needed help with my swimming costume. I'd shuffle out of the change rooms trying, unfortunately unsuccessfully, to hide my matchstick thin body. Next I'd be strapped into a mechanical chair at the pool's edge and lowered into a warm, swimming pool. How I hated that chair! Sitting in it, my crookedness utterly revealed by a swimming costume, I couldn't deny or escape my pitiful physical appearance.

What further humiliations awaited me? A year ago I was a grade-school teacher, with a car, an apartment, friends—*sans souci*. A year ago my biggest problems were romantic. Now, at 24, I was a twisted skeleton in a wheelchair. When the hunky young physiotherapist smiled at me he didn't see an attractive woman—only a distorted patient. The thought hurt.

The physio instructed me to do slow leg movements back and forth in the warm water. It gave me relief, but that was short-lived. It was replaced by acute anxiety about how I was going to get out of the pool and how I'd dress myself. Standing half naked, waiting for Mum to dress me was embarrassing so I'd always start trying to dress myself. Usually my wrists were too sore and weak to hold a towel to dry my body. Feeling defeated I would call for help. As Mum wiped me down I'd feel like I was her little girl again. However, the comforting thought was all too brief. I knew what was coming next. Getting my bathers off was a major effort and stressed me out. They were wet and stuck to my skin so I needed even more strength to get them off. As I tried to pull them down they'd roll. I'd end up crying in frustration and Mum would usually pull them off for me. She'd crouch down and hold my knickers open for me, while I leaned on her back and tried to lift my leg high enough off the ground to step into them. Being naked at this age in front of my Mum never felt right, I was awkward and self-conscious. Hydrotherapy was fast becoming another task that frustrated and exhausted me and made me angry.

I didn't want to live this life anymore and it was clear that something had to change. The trial therapy prescribed by Dr Reisman had not worked. I guessed that my disease was too aggressive.

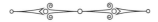

Mum and I went to Dr Reisman's consulting rooms together for my second consultation. Dad was not with us this time. What we heard, in crisp medical terms, neither cheered us nor left us entirely without hope.

'Karen, your rheumatoid factor is strongly positive and your blood count shows inflammation. I feel you need to go on a disease-suppressive agent today. It may take between four and six weeks to actually start working and rashes and mouth ulcers may occur. There's also the rare possibility of drug-induced hepatitis and, very rarely, bone marrow suppression. You'll have to have regular supervision and blood tests. There are no guarantees and this drug works in about 60 per cent of people with RA. Come back in December and we'll see how you're doing.'

Being back on a regime of drugs made me feel like I had failed and let everyone down, especially Mum and Mrs Hills. A few days after visiting Dr Reisman a letter arrived from Mrs Hills.

> *Never think that you are not going to get better—you will Karen—negative thoughts are soul destroying. Keep on with your treatment, keep on praying, keep on hoping, you will emerge with a strong spirit, willing and able to fulfill any work to help others that you are destined for.*
> *Till I hear from you, God bless you.*
> *Margaret x*

It was only four months since I had left her clinic. How could I ever tell her I'd failed?

14 November: Once again I am thrust into the throes of confusion. Natural therapies have not worked for me. I've read every book I can find on alternative medicine. Another matronly nurse has eliminated everything else from my diet. Now I can only eat a few fruits, a few vegetables and millet seed—which they feed to birds. It seems like almost everybody is saying I have allergies to almost every food. I've now been bed-ridden for weeks and am completely dependent on Mum for everything again. The visits to Dr Reisman haven't done enough to help. My mind is crazed. There's no sanity to all this and there's no peace in my body, my mind or my life anymore. I think I am at rock bottom. I am a prisoner in this damn apartment and I'm tired of being carried up and down 48 stairs. I had to have my knees aspirated again. I'm so tired and scared that this disease will just keep getting worse. My fears are beginning to attack me as much as the disease.

Dear God, please give me the strength to cope with this and show me how to be grateful for what I do have. I have learned about how precious life is, how amazing my support network is and what life is like for the disabled and the old. I am thankful for that.

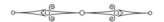

One day a letter arrived from the government benefits office notifying me that it was time to assess my status. On the appointed date Mum drove me to a low-slung, brown brick building near the railway line in Hurstville. In the government offices we sat amongst pensioners, the disabled of all ages and brazen dole-moochers—fit young cads who surfed all day and collected government handouts that kept them in beers and board wax. I looked around the waiting room, my stomach in knots. Were these my new peers? Was I to spend the rest of my life among the halt and the lame, the aged and the ne'er-do-wells of the world? I was only 24 years old. In the Bible, God gave us three score years and ten. I would be satisfied with nothing less.

The administrator assigned to my case, a balding guy in a striped tie, asked me a few questions, checked out the doctor's report, ruffled the pages in my file, then pushed his eye-glasses on to his shiny brow and pronounced me unfit for work. Ever!

The words flew from his mouth like a barrage of insults.

'Your disease is very aggressive and there is much deformity in one so young. I do not anticipate that your condition will improve a great deal so I am going to recommend that you be put on an invalid pension.'

I was now being permanently placed out of the workforce. There was, officially, no prospect of me ever being capable of working again. All hope evaporated. I had hit rock bottom. Before I was back in Mum's car I'd already decided to prove him wrong. A desire to fight back bombarded my thoughts.

'I can't go on an invalid pension when I am only in my twenties! I won't let them label me like that.'

And so my spiritual fight began. My RA was not going to beat up my body as well as my soul! I turned to Mum and sobbed: 'I won't let them put me on an invalid pension.'

Mum had not heard me talk like this before. I was determined and focused. And so my new journey began. It was time to return from the abyss.

Chapter 5
Back in Black

It was spring 1989 and I was back on oral cortisone, anti-inflammatory drugs and immune system suppressants. I took my trusty meds morning and night and never looked back.

Yes, I knew my pills weren't *healing* me; once RA had a secure foothold, the best you can hope for is slow degeneration of the joints with minimal pain. But after my all-natural months at Margaret Hills' Clinic in England and home in Australia at Mum's apartment, that sounded like a pretty good deal.

When I was strong enough I moved into a big, three-bedroom house in Lugarno on the northern shores of the Georges River some 20 kilometres (12 miles) south of Sydney. Margo, together with one of the glamour girls from the European trip and a pilot friend, joined me in converting one of the living areas into a bedroom. We split the rent four ways.

Lugarno is an affluent suburb with large areas of natural bush land, rolling hills and parks. Having been brought up in Melbourne, I didn't have a wide knowledge of the outer suburbs of Sydney. I had first heard of Lugarno during the 1983 Ash Wednesday bushfires which burnt through hundreds of thousands of hectares of land in Australia's south east. These disastrous wild fires, caused by extreme temperatures and hot northerly winds, spread quickly through three Australian states—South Australia, Victoria and New South Wales.

With the move to a new home came a glow of happiness—for the first time in some years. Lisa had returned from overseas and my life began to feel somewhat normal. Weekends were spent watching and learning about Rugby, the dominant football code in NSW, and enjoying a few ales at the local rugby club.

The Lugarno house was not the best choice for me physically, but I didn't care. It rested on the side of a precipitous slope and was spread over three levels with lots of stairs. The driveway was steep and challenging. Mum, worried about how I would cope, tried to convince me I needed a house with no steps. We had lived together for nearly two years, bumping along over the rockiest road of my life to date and, with the improvement in my health, I couldn't wait to be free.

Mum also needed her space. She had centred her world around me for far too long and I understood that she had to move forward. She never admitted that to me but I sensed it. When I told her it was time for me to move out I knew she was relieved. We both understood there was nothing more she could do for me.

Our new home quickly gained a reputation as 'the party house'. Guys from the local rugby club, Southern Districts, would drop in at all hours of the night, or we'd come home and find them asleep on the doorstep or on balconies outside the girls' rooms.

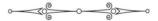

Steve's life had also moved forward. He took me to lunch one day and told me he and Trudy were to be married.

'She makes me happy and I know she'll be a good mum one day.'

I was pleased for him—Trudy was kind and compassionate. At times when I was suffering she had rubbed my feet and helped my mother out in her role as my carer. Above all, if my brother was happy then so was I.

With Steve getting married and Mum dating again it felt like my family, already restructured by the divorce, was changing once more. This was unsettling. I had some moments when I feared being alone and getting sick again, but I blocked them out and tried to focus on the present. I felt lucky to be well enough to be able to mingle with my friends and to rediscover the young woman who had once lived in my battered body.

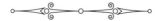

Dad had his own problems in Melbourne. The 1989 pilots' dispute was in full swing and the Australian Federation of Airline Pilots clashed head-on with airline management which was backed by the tenacious Prime Minister, Bob Hawke. The boldness of the founding fathers of aviation in our desolate country—like Sir Charles Kingsford Smith after whom Sydney Airport is named—and their brash pioneering spirit had helped build a debonair image of pilots in the minds of the Australian public. This rubbed off on me. I was proud to be an aviator's daughter. But the clash between employers and employees in the aviation industry was about to change this popular—and to me, cherished—image.

The dispute caused disruption not only to flights across Australia, but also to tourism and many related businesses and cast the pilots in a poor light. The press and the public toppled them off their pedestal, accusing them of, amongst other things, constantly being on strike over holiday periods. To crown it all they were dubbed *glorified bus drivers*.

Eventually, in response to common law actions filed by airline employers, the pilots resigned *en masse*. Dad was part of the collective resignation. He had worked for Australian Airlines (TAA) for 36 years and now his flying days were over. They were gone in the blink of an eye. There was no golden handshake; no 'thank you'—just the boot. Dad's decision not to return to work as so-called scab labour and to remain in his home country rather than take a job flying for an overseas airline marked the end of his aviation career. Understandably, he had difficulties reconciling himself to his new situation so, during the times we spent together, we'd often focus on his problems rather than mine.

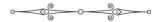

During my first weeks in the Lugarno house I tried to build up muscles that had withered like unwatered roses over the past few years. Hydro and heat therapy filled my days. My general health had improved considerably and at least some of my quality of life had been restored. I was acutely aware, however, that the pain and deformities were hiding in the wings, masked on a daily basis by my doses of cortisone. Hanging over my head like a perpetual thundercloud was the knowledge that my disease was ever-present and, just to make sure I didn't forget, it delivered constant reminders.

Despite my new medication regimen, doing simple things still presented difficulties. Standing to watch a game of football or raising a glass of wine to my mouth were all challenges. I tackled every hurdle that stood in my way as I was as determined to overcome these problems as I was to restore my dignity in the bathroom. Little by little, day by day things started to get easier.

In a letter to my general practitioner Dr Reisman wrote:

I have reviewed Karen a couple of times since I last wrote to you. Things do appear to be improving. She has reduced her Prednisone (oral cortisone) to 1 mg per day, but has continued with Dolobid 500 mg, Plaquenil 200 mg per day and Salzopyrin. She is troubled by pain in the left second MTP joint (where the big toe meets the foot) but happily there was no soft tissue swelling in that joint.

Her major problem is pain in the right hip and there was certainly crepitus (grating) in the right hip, loss of movement and joint space. X-rays revealed this destruction. I therefore had a lengthy chat with Karen about her right hip and advised her that we should try to delay hip replacement as long as possible, particularly because she is only 25. I encouraged her to continue with her hydrotherapy and exercise program.

Clinically her rheumatoid appears to be in remission and I have asked her to continue with the above-mentioned medications.

We also had a chat again about pregnancy and I felt that the question of hip replacement prior to any planned pregnancy in a few years time should be reviewed closer to that date. I feel that we probably shouldn't replace the hip solely to facilitate a vaginal delivery. I feel the indication should really be pain and limitation of function.

I have asked her to return for periodic review.

After rebuilding and strengthening my wasted muscles with

workouts and gaining more mobility with water exercise and heat therapy, I applied for a position as a first-grade teacher at a nearby school.

Would the thin, balding principal of St Luke's Catholic School sign me up if he knew I had RA? I decided I couldn't risk telling him about my problem. At the conclusion of the interview with this kindly headmaster I turned to him and made an appeal that, in retrospect, may have puzzled him:

'All I want is to be given a chance. Thank you for interviewing me.'

I was appointed to the Grade One position.

My spirits soared. Once again I felt that I could fly. Despite the government's conclusion that I was an invalid—and its generous offer of handouts for the rest of my days—I wanted to work. I wanted the feelings of self-worth and satisfaction that come with a pay cheque. And I missed teaching. I needed to be back in a classroom, where problems can be puzzled out with patience and encouragement, where anger can be transformed with words and where happiness, joy, generosity and love are part of every day. My pay cheque also delivered the independence that I so desperately needed and, even though it was a struggle, I could afford to pay the rent.

So I was back in the workforce, doing what I loved, for the first time in nearly two and a half years. I had renewed freedom. I felt happy and fortunate and my confidence started to grow. Welcome weight crept back on my gaunt frame and I even allowed myself to date again.

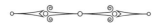

In December of that year, 1989, I met Paul. He came into my life as fast and unexpectedly as Melbourne's changeable weather. Margo had met him in Honolulu and reconnected with him when she arrived home. She introduced us one summer Sunday afternoon at a local beachside bar. From the east coast to the west coast, Sunday sessions are a tradition in Australia. Paul's tanned, glowing skin and carved biceps showed themselves off in his Bonds T-shirt. More than six feet tall, with hush-puppy eyes, he was so handsome that he couldn't help but stand out from the crowd. He sang and played the guitar and captivated the females in the audience. I was attracted to him like a magnet—just like every other girl in the bar. I couldn't believe it when he came over to chat to Margo and hung around to get to know me. Paul came home with me to Lugarno that night and our relationship bloomed.

It would become a five-year-long liaison—but it would also bore a hole in the relationship I had been trying to rebuild with my mother. Once again I resisted any criticisms and told myself I had quite the catch.

After being so sick in my early twenties, I believed I had now found all I ever wanted. I had regained enough of my health to function— or at least to give the impression of being the ever-elusive 'normal'. As well, I was teaching and sharing a house with my girlfriends and it felt like I was falling in love. After being without these things for so long I felt that I could finally move from just existing to living again and on to actually enjoying life.

On the surface Paul was every girl's dream. He would write me songs or make tapes of his favorite sentimental lyrics and give them to me, or have the music ready to play in the car when I hopped in. In the early days of our relationship I would come home to find roses on my bed, handmade cards and framed pictures of us. He was Mr Romantic. Everything in my life was great. My journal reads:

> He really cares. He's gentle, genuine and thoughtful and doesn't live for the guys.

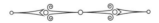

My first year with Paul was wonderful. I felt as if he had put an end to all my suffering. I aligned myself with him and he did the same with me. We had fun. I was truly content from the inside out for the first time in 10 years.

It seemed like my arthritis was a 'non issue' with Paul, especially since it was under reasonable control. My life felt uncomplicated and very good. Through my disease I had learned to appreciate the gift of 'normalcy' and to be grateful for the simple things in life. Dad had always told me to do that. He said to me often: 'I am a simple man, I like simple things. And they don't have to cost much to make me happy.'

I never quite understood what he meant until I lost my ability to do basic things effortlessly. So even if it meant that I had to continue to be on horrendous amounts of medication, the trade-off was worth it.

Paul, however, was a restless soul and within 12 months he had grown tired of what he suddenly called our 'humdrum' relationship. The excitement of the early days of discovering each other were over and we'd settled into a routine. To him I was security. I represented the sanctity of a home and a place to relax away from his sometimes stressful family life with his Mum and Dad.

I too had my private worries but refused to admit them—even to myself. Paul had a bungalow out the back of his parents' home and I was not comfortable visiting him there. I saw frightening similarities between Paul and my previous boyfriend, Geoff. Both of them had been raised by parents who drank and smoked far too much. It wasn't until much later that I realised how important it was to match the values you have been raised to believe in to your partner's values.

Paul needed his ego stroked. Even though he was in a so-called committed relationship with me, he still wanted to be pursued by other women. The feeling excited him and made him feel like a real Aussie bloke.

He stopped writing me songs and singing to me on the bedside. His boredom and discontent with our life manifested itself in moods that swung back and forth like a pendulum.

Unwilling to break the spell he'd cast on me and unwilling to get in touch with my new reality and let go of my dreams, I began to take responsibility for his happiness. I thought I could make him happy and make him feel good if only I did more. I started to respond to his every need like I was his mistress not his girlfriend. Though Paul never laid a hand on me, the parallels between him and Geoff were becoming alarmingly clear. He lacked ambition and drive. And then there were his addictions, which were well hidden behind the music and, in the beginning, the intensity of a new romance. Being with Paul was just like being with Geoff—but I refused to do anything about it. RA had again trapped me in a relationship that was far from perfect because I felt too inadequate and fearful to set boundaries.

It wasn't until our relationship got serious and I moved from the Lugarno house and into another southern suburb with Paul that I had a true indication of just how bad his drinking addiction was. Paul handled all of life's problems with alcohol. My decision to move in with him—in a rented house in the small, tree-lined suburb of Hurstville Grove—was unimportant to my family and friends. They all had their lives to live—my family was 'getting on with it'; Margo had moved back home and the 'glamour sister' was now married. The pilot with whom we lived with took over the lease and off I went. No-one was worried. Paul had hidden his habits well.

Hurstville Grove had the ambience of a village and our new home was surrounded by bushland and backed on to a huge park. At first glance the house looked good, but it was constructed of weatherboard (wood panels) and was damp to the core. The sunlight couldn't penetrate through the trees and condensation clung to the walls.

My health began to deteriorate and Paul started to spend more and more time away from home—at the pub. In the beginning, I thought it was because of me, the fault of my illness and its inherent pressure. It wasn't long before things began to spiral out of control. A quick drink on the way home from work led to later and later nights, then weekends when he just didn't come home.

I've always wondered if stress triggers disease. For me, it seemed there was a correlation. Before long, my medications stopped working and once again, I began to feel as if I was losing control of my body and of my RA. My doctor decided to put me on a very aggressive drug called Methotrexate. It was considered to be a breakthrough drug for the treatment of RA in the 1980s. It was also used to treat certain types of cancer. I was told to watch for a long list of side effects including include hair loss, infections, impairment of fertility and lung disease.

On 6 September 1991 Dr Reisman wrote:

Clearly, Karen's current regime is not adequately controlling her rheumatoid and I therefore asked her to recommence Methotrexate 2.5 mg. This has been ceased previously with Karen because of dizziness… I do not think this was solely related to the Methotrexate and so I feel it is worth the risk of recommencing this drug. It does seem to be the most potent of all rheumatoid drugs. I have outlined all the side effects. I will of course arrange for regular haematological supervision.

I have asked Karen to return for review in another couple of weeks to assess progress.

It seemed like Methotrexate truly was a last resort medication because of its potential toxic reactions. I didn't believe I had a choice. I wasn't responding to other less potent classes of RA drugs any more. Again the choice was for quality of life. By going on Methotrexate I believed I'd taken the steps I needed to take control of my disease and to not end up in a wheelchair.

I made my own decisions with my medications now and told Mum and Dad what I had decided to do rather than asking them for advice.

Next I took action to try to get my relationship with Paul back on track. I became obsessed with the idea that I had to fix things with him even if it was damaging to my own self. Keeping the peace and making him happy meant everything to me. I became a martyr. When I heard the car door slam in the drive I would try to anticipate his mood. I walked on egg shells. I vowed not to comment if he was late or 'agro' for no reason. I wanted this relationship to work. Paul was the man who had made me whole again and I defined my 'new' self by being with him.

Somehow, I convinced myself this relationship was what I needed, but I couldn't get the same amount of control over my body. This was no surprise really. My body never did what I wanted it to do anyway. It reacted to the stress. I had butterflies in my stomach all the time, my heart would race and my palms would be clammy. I was a bundle of nerves.

I told no-one about my home life, not my brother, not my mum and dad and not my closest friends. I wanted to keep my sadness to myself because I hoped we could figure it out together. I knew from my experience with Geoff that unsolicited advice from family and friends did more to sabotage a situation than to help it.

Eventually, I understood there were patterns to Paul's mood swings; certain times of the year emerged as red flag months. Boys' weekends, daily intoxication and spending sprees filled the months from September until January. It all began with the end of the football season. Then the rampage would really start. Weeks of abstinence leading up to the finals would be followed by extreme weekends of binge drinking. Time and again I'd hear: 'It's the culture. That's what Aussie blokes do.'

Footballers' wives and girlfriends all around Australia accept this attitude because they have no choice. There is an unquestioning culture that comes with the sport. The footballers feel entitled to behave like this. The subject is closed because the boys will do it anyway. And when the whole football team is binge drinking it somehow seems more acceptable. By saying something to your partner you risk looking like the ogre; the difficult 'wife' who won't give her husband a 'leave pass'. So you just don't go there.

Binge drinking the night after a game was just the beginning. Expecting to hear from Paul before Sunday afternoon was also foolish. Footballers' wives and girlfriends were wise to have low expectations. It took me many sleepless nights and many weekends to learn that. I often lay in bed waiting to hear the car door slam closed. My lack of sleep and the damp house also helped trigger my RA to flare. When Paul finally arrived home, sometimes on a Monday morning, he'd be cranky for the rest of the week. Even though I knew what to expect because of Geoff, I never remembered him going 'absent without leave' for weekends at a time. I blamed myself. I also tried to understand the void that footballers feel when the footy season finishes; with no training and less interaction with their mates it was all that some of them needed to send them over the edge. The phone calls from old team mates would start on a Thursday night and then the binge drinking cycle would begin again.

A few weeks after the last game, the end-of-season footy trip would roll around. Bali and Hawaii were always popular destinations and I knew of single girls who would book their trips just because they knew these were their much-loved players' haunts. While Paul was away on his trip one year some balloons arrived. I was thrilled, thinking that Paul's romantic side had returned.

The card read: 'Meeting you the other night was wonderful. Please call me.' I knew I was losing him.

After the players returned from their footy trips the Spring Racing Carnival would be in full swing and it would begin all over again. Then there was Christmas, New Year and Australia Day. They were all excuses to binge drink. Paul could get instant gratification through drinking, gambling and flirting with random women. I didn't set enough boundaries and his actions became increasingly erratic, darting from manic highs to ominous lows.

Thursday was also payday and this was when he was at his moodiest. He usually went straight from work as a swimming pool technician to the pub. Sometimes I'd get in my car and drive to all the local pubs in search of his work van—and him. I'd find him all pumped up, sitting on a scratched bar stool playing the 'pokies', waiting for an elusive row of cherries, or aces or whatever hit the jackpot on that particular slot machine. His reaction at my appearance was never welcoming so I would leave. When he finally stumbled home, his mood was entirely dependent on whether he'd won or lost his pay cheque. For months I had no idea that the trigger for his mood swings was losing money. I thought it was all about me and that the pub was a way of escaping from 'us'.

Strangely, I didn't have a clue he was addicted to gambling, nor did I see his drinking as bingeing. I kept on blaming myself and my disease for all of our problems—that was probably easier for me than to face his addictions and the possibility of being alone. I didn't know it, but my fear of being alone was dominating me and becoming an obstacle as big as the disease itself. I made excuses for Paul. Lots of excuses. And I tried to fix everything. I was my mother's daughter.

On the day after New Year's Day, in 1991, I copied this poem by an unknown author into my journal as a reminder of how to be a better person:

Let me be a little kinder
Just a little bit more blinder
To the faults of those around me
Let me praise a little more
Let me be when I am weary,
Just a little cheerie
Think a little more of others

And a little less of me.

I thought if I became a better person, a nicer person we'd be okay. It worked for a while—but I couldn't hide the truth from my journal. Towards the end of 1991 I wrote about the troubles that faced me.

19 November: Our problems seem to start at this time of the year, except things are worse because now we're engaged! It happened a few months ago. Paul didn't make it an especially memorable night, but we celebrated at a restaurant with both families. His actions have been a bit strange since. Paul asked Dad to buy the engagement ring while he was on a trip to Hawaii. Paul said they were cheaper there. Dad bought the ring, but Paul didn't have the cash to pay him. Now he is paying Dad off, $30 bucks a week. I know Dad doesn't mind; he thinks he is helping. Mum and Dad seem happy for me. They just want to see me in a good marriage, just like Steve. If only they knew what's really been going on. The truth is a future with Paul is now scaring me. If I am completely honest, we've had two years of on and off problems. I don't think he knows what he wants. He thinks he wants me but he doesn't; he wants to settle down but he doesn't, he wants money but sometimes he couldn't care less about it. Now he's not talking to me and I keep pushing for him to open up which makes him even more distant. What hurts the most is that he said he can't touch me because of my RA.

I say I understand, but I don't. It hurts. He also said he doesn't want to touch me because he doesn't *feel* that way. That's the real truth! I'm now scared to touch him for fear he'll reject me. I'm tired of looking at his back in bed. I think his love for me is a *feeling sorry kind a love*. If this is true, I don't want it.

1 December: I am beginning to notice that I have 'tummy fear' a lot of the time when Paul and I are together. My stomach is full of butterflies and I am constantly nervous because I don't know what to expect. Perhaps I need to listen to my body's reaction more. Paul has been trying harder. At least he is touching me now, but that probably won't last. He is still going out with the boys but now it's on Tuesday nights. I get to be with him during 'prime time' on the weekends. Lucky me! I am also beginning to feel like we have no financial security because we have nothing. I do not even know if he is saving for a life together after the wedding. Isn't planning for the future part of getting married and that means saving?

18 December: After I wrote my last diary entry Paul didn't come home. As I tossed and turned in our bed that long night I decided that he'd pushed me too far. I would postpone our wedding. When he finally arrived home the next day I told him I didn't want to be married in April. He has been in the *I am so sorry mode* ever since but his behaviour is convincing me that nothing has changed. I worry that I am staying with Paul only because of my fears about being alone and of finding love again—because of my disease.

It didn't take long for Paul's gambling addiction to escalate. But even when he created chaos, I preferred to ignore it. In truth his withdrawal from me and his mood swings were not because of me—or my disease. It was gambling that dictated where Paul went—and when he stayed at home it was not because he was happy and content to be with me, it was because he had lost all his money to the poker machines at the pub.

He continued to let his addictions debilitate him and I continued to let my neediness debilitate me. I just couldn't leave him and pass up the chance that our relationship might still work. I continued to dream about walking down the aisle.

But try as I might I never reached the altar in my dream.

Chapter 6
Darling of the Universe

Soft is the rain that falls upon the flowers in your garden
They grow in vain for the one that isn't here
We can't have heaven without the dying
Sometimes it just makes me feel like crying
And I felt for a second
I was the only one in this world
Then an angel did tell me
You were the darling of the universe
You knew it well before your time
There was no shame no pretending
I'm not so sure I could wear that brave a face.
Darling of the Universe – Mark Lizotte
(Lyrics printed with permisson of EMI Publishing Lizard Songs)

It was New Year's Eve. A group of friends, good music and a happy crowd—this was all I needed to usher in 1992. Even before the party began I felt exhausted. I was fighting a cold which, like an unwelcome relative, had hung around for about three months. My local doctor had prescribed antibiotics a few days before Christmas in the hope that they would work their magic and clear it up. But still I felt sluggish—tired like an infant being taken to bed after falling asleep in the back seat of a car.

We had chosen to eat at a Thai restaurant where the décor was plain and simple. The aromas from the food made me feel sick. I didn't eat.

Later, at the Cock-n-Bull Tavern in Bondi Junction I stared at the hands of my watch. The place was packed with English tourists and locals. The crowd was singing and dancing. There was a good vibe but I couldn't get into it. Last year, to be out in Bondi with Paul would have been the ultimate New Year's Eve for me. But I had grown tired of the arrogance and the party tricks of some of his friends. They'd smuggled small bottles of spirits down the front of their trousers into the pub and then stolen fluorescent lights from the men's toilets. Perhaps it could have been funny if I'd been drinking. Some of Paul's Aussie Rules football-playing mates were the same ones who had led him astray; so for me the joke had long been over.

Finally, the time on my watch said 12.10 a.m. New Year's Eve was finished, we were into New Year's Day and I wanted to make a quick exit.

'Being out with you is like being out with my grandma,' grumbled Paul, belittling me in front of his mates.

I was too sick to care so I told him I was leaving.

'If you want a ride home with me you'd better come now.'

Bondi Junction to Hurstville was quite a distance—an expensive cab fare—so he conceded and we left together. He was too drunk to argue.

Somehow I had made it home, but I was feeling very ill indeed. Paul crashed on to our bed in a drunken stupor. He was comatose.

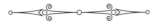

My temperature began to rise. I was experiencing hot sweats then cold sweats in confusing repetition. I shook Paul to tell him I needed help.

Afterwards I could not believe that I did not call an ambulance myself. I really don't know why I didn't. Perhaps I had slipped into a state of 'co-dependence', or perhaps I was not coherent enough to understand that I could call for help myself. I have no idea. I do know that I'd gotten into a habit of fighting my body when it was sick, of not reading warning signs and of picking myself up and brushing myself off. Perhaps that was why, or perhaps it was more of a laissez-faire feeling—being aware of the problem but not wanting to do anything about it. This experience was indeed a lesson for me and one that I will remember all my life. Ultimately, we are all responsible for ourselves especially in matters of health.

'Paul, I can't breathe properly…I can't breathe. Wake up, please wake up.' My pleas went unanswered as Paul snored on.

I was gasping for every breath. The night seemed to go on and on forever. The hands of the clock seemed to stop still. I was saturated with perspiration. Finally, as the first light of dawn lit up our bedroom window Paul stirred from his alcohol-induced sleep.

'Paul, I'm really sick, I need to go to the hospital. You have to take me now. Don't call my family. I don't want them to worry.'

I knew there was nothing they could do at that moment. Steve was on an overseas trip, Dad was in Perth for the New Year and Mum was on the Central Coast.

In the early hours of New Year's Day Paul drove me to St George Hospital. Finally, I was behind the starched curtain in the emergency ward. I felt glad to be there. I felt safe. I lay on the rigid bed, half listening to stories of New Year's Eve revellers who had come to grief and ended up needing medical help. Not long after I arrived I was admitted into a hospital ward. Every breath was still a huge effort. I knew I didn't have much left to give. My vision was myopic; my body was shaking and I started hallucinating. On the opposite side of the hospital room I saw a horde of naked mannequins on an empty bed. Then they were all over the place. They were opposite me, at the end of the bed, next to the bed, to the left of me and to my right. They were driving me crazy. My mind was abuzz. Doctors began to surround my bed, but they were a blur too. I closed my eyes and tried to listen to what they were saying.

'It's bilateral pneumonia. She's hallucinating because of a lack of oxygen. Give her an oxygen mask and see if you can get her to tell you who to call. Her boyfriend's left.'

Trish, a mother of three and a work colleague from St Luke's was my first choice. She came to the hospital straight after she received the call. She'd mentored me at work and I often talked to her about my problems with Paul. When Trish arrived at the hospital and saw me wearing an oxygen mask and gasping for each breath she made her own decision to call Mum.

Just as I was being transferred to the intensive care unit (ICU) Mum arrived from the Central Coast. My bed, the nurses, doctors and Paul, who had been called back to the hospital because of the ICU transfer, filled the space in the elevator. There was no room for my mother. As the elevator doors shut her out, I saw a look of desperation in her eyes that I will never forget. I understood that it was her place to be there next to me and not Paul's. It was wrong of Paul to have taken up her space and I needed my mum not him.

In the ICU I was hooked up to all kinds of monitors. A young, male nurse who smelled like he smoked, attached sticky round adhesives in strategic positions on my body. Cords were inserted into silver holes in the adhesives. The machine attached to the cords was not unlike a portable television. A green line beeped across the screen. Clear fluids hung from bags on hooks. As I floated in and out of consciousness I could hear the doctors talking about performing a tracheotomy—an incision into my windpipe so that oxygen could be delivered to my lungs more quickly. Mum wanted to know if there was 'any other way'. A slightly overweight female doctor replied.

'The fluid is building in her lungs. We need to dry that up and monitor her liquids. We can try her with oxygen treatment and restrict her liquids to a few droplets of water on her lips every hour. She'll have to wear a large mask and we will be filling the lungs with hot air. If this doesn't work we'll have to do the tracheotomy.'

A 'long line' was inserted into a vein in my arm and fed through to my chest. A simple intravenous line in the forearm wouldn't be good enough. My veins might collapse. I guess they figured I'd be there for a while. Inserting the long line was bearable, but after a short time I started having severe pain in my chest. It was as if a knife was being thrust in and out. The nurses took the line out and began again.

In brief moments of clarity I wondered whether pneumonia was going to be my worst enemy rather than the RA I'd been trying to fight for so long. Every breath became a battle for my life but I felt strangely peaceful. Though I did not want to die, I knew I wasn't scared of dying either. It was seeing the fear in Mum's eyes that made me want to live. Her eyes were strong yet frail; hopeful yet afraid. They told the story of a mother's sacrifice—love and pain. There had been so much of that with us.

Mum's blue eyes, looking at me from the base of my bed, gave me the strength I needed to *will* myself to live. I saw her distress and wanted to fight just like that day we were in the government office. I knew I wasn't ready to say goodbye.

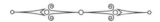

'Where are you, Dad, where are you? Why aren't you here yet? Are you on your way?' I mumbled this question many times over during my disturbed consciousness. I was aware of Dad's absence and Mum's presence, but I genuinely thought he'd be on his way and that's all that mattered.

I didn't know that Dad was stuck in Perth unable to get a flight back to the east coast during the holiday season. I convinced myself that Dad couldn't have known how sick I was otherwise he would have been there. Somehow, someway he would have been there. So I wasn't angry. I knew it was 'just Dad'. I didn't stop to think that Mum was alone again, unable to share her pain with my father.

I spent 14 days in the ICU—and because of that, my life would be forever changed. I was momentarily a part of another world where people were struggling to hold on to life. It was a flash of time, just a snapshot that was all, but it was a lesson I needed to learn. My lot in life didn't seem that bad anymore, even with RA. Who was it who said everything was relative?

Luke lay in the next ICU bed. He'd wrapped his new Christmas toy, a brand new Holden ute he'd been given by his parents, around a tree. He was in a coma. His family visited every day and played 'Oh What a Wonderful World' over and over again. It was his favourite song. On the back of a torn envelope I scribbled a note to remind me of those first weeks of 1992.

10 January: Luke's dad just came to visit his son. Luke hasn't moved since I saw him admitted. Surrounded by despair, heartache, hope and anxiety his dad still found the time to show love for someone else—me. 'How are you today, Karen?' he quietly asked.

'Okay,' I replied weakly.

But my mind was having a dialogue of its own. What a man he must be to even bother to ask! Then he told me he broke down yesterday for the first time since Luke's car accident. He said he went to his mum's and cried.

Dear God, I pray that Luke will have the gift of life given back to him and that his parents' vigil and suffering may end soon.

The nurses and doctors on any ICU ward deserve a medal. A couple of people died during my time in intensive care. How hard it must be to be assigned to a case that just doesn't make it. I knew they were told to remain detached, but I could see in their eyes how hard that was.

After two weeks in the ICU I was back at home in Hurstville Grove. I was one of the lucky ones. My recovery from pneumonia was swift in the end and the nurses said that they had never seen anyone discharged directly from the ICU before—most patients went to other wards to regain their health before leaving the hospital. They found it amusing.

Paul's feelings towards me had changed while I was in hospital. I could read it in his manner. I knew I looked terrible and that didn't help. I was even thinner than before and I had dry sores all around my mouth from the oxygen mask. I decided there was nothing I could do to improve the situation so I remained quiet.

My time in the ICU had become another of the pivotal moments that I experienced in my life. I had watched Luke fight and hang on to his life and I'd learned from my own battle to save mine. This gave me a calm, inner strength that I had not had before. The last I heard of Luke was that he was doing better. Before I was released from the ICU he was moved to a high dependency ward. His eyes had opened and he was conscious but still unable to speak or move. I often wonder about where he is today and whether he can walk.

When I was fully recovered, I decided to move out of the Hurstville Grove house that I shared with Paul and to take a room in the home of Lisa's father, Jack, in Mortdale.

Jack loved our family, he understood my disease and his home was close to the school where I was teaching. He was one of those family friends you call Uncle even though they are not related. Mum had maintained the friendship through the years and Jack had always been there for us all. Lisa had returned to the States—chasing love—but was happy that I had moved into her father's home. Jack and Lisa's mum were divorced and over the years he'd welcomed his niece, me, my brother and various other Qantas pilots into his home. It was a place where we could stay until we got on our feet in Sydney.

The Mortdale house and Jack represented so much more to me than just a place to hang my hat. It was a haven of comfort, security and childhood memories. Everything there was exactly as I had remembered it as a little girl. The 1970s bird wallpaper covered every niche in the master bedroom, the trundle bed that I used to sleep on in Lisa's room was in its place and the souvenirs from our shared family holidays were scattered around the living areas.

Being at 37A Kemp Street also brought back memories of happier days in Mum and Dad's marriage. On one occasion they travelled overseas for six weeks without Steve and me. They took us out of our schools in Melbourne and enrolled us at the Sydney schools of Lisa and her brother Mark so we could be secure while they were away.

Jack was a selfless man and I loved him dearly. While I stayed with him after leaving Paul he did lots of thoughtful things for me—like picking up dinner on the way home, opening the lids of things I could not manage and washing my car.

Paul accepted my decision to move in with Jack. I think he was even relieved. He moved closer to the footy club and into a house full of footballers. We kept dating.

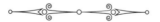

Every teacher keeps close to his or her heart stories of the children they'll never forget. I met my first unforgettable student while at St Luke's—a bright-eyed spitfire named Amy whose physical and intellectual limitations were surpassed by an indomitable spirit. Amy had Down's Syndrome. Mainstreamed into my first-grade class, she threw herself into all of our activities and though she faced greater challenges than her classmates, she became their leader.

I will never forget Amy's first day in Grade One. Her smile beamed across the crowded room of 32 infants. She was proudly dressed in her brand-new checkered summer uniform. Her hair was swept either side of her face in plaits which were fastened with perfectly formed blue bows. Her mum, Colleen, stood quietly at the classroom door as, after the summer break, Amy happily greeted old friends from her kindergarten year. Colleen looked at me with a smile and said, with a certain amount of pride: 'She likes to be boss.'

Colleen was a nurse assisting at Amy's delivery. After her parents discovered that Amy was a 'Downs' baby they put her up for adoption. It was a wise choice by her biological parents who knew they would not be able to cope. Colleen was a devoted single mother who loved Amy as if she were her own.

Amy and I quickly became friends. A typical exchange between us:

'Amy, would you like me to help you with your letters?'

'I don't need help.'

'How about if I sit next to you and guide your hand as you write?'

'I can do it, Miss Ager. I'll show you.'

Amy showed me many things, including her uncanny empathy. My disease was very active that year and I was struggling to hide my symptoms. Some mornings Amy would look into my eyes, reach for my hand and begin stroking it gently. During story-reading time, she planted herself on the rug directly in front of me—in 'her spot'—and would quietly slip off my shoes and start massaging my aching feet. She read my emotions about Paul with stunning accuracy. Her hugs always had extra gusto on the days Paul and I had been fighting.

Amy even joked with the children about her colostomy bag.

When Amy was born, like many other children with Down's Syndrome, some of her internal organs were not fully developed.

Amy had digestive tract issues—an undeveloped peristaltic action meant that her intestine would become blocked. So she had a colostomy bag. Her bag often filled up in class and needed to be emptied. On occasions it burst open. We were all fine with this. Amy would make a joke about it and the other kids would try to help. I didn't have an assistant to lend a hand with Amy, but all I had to do was log a quick call to Colleen and she'd be there in a flash.

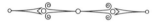

In Australia, regular elementary, or primary school teachers, are required to teach physical education (PE). Any kind of sport, however, was out of the question for me. I let gym slip—I'm not proud to admit it—scheduling one class per week, tops, and assigning activities that I could monitor without demonstrating or participating, like obstacle courses. With a clipboard on my arm, I'd observe my students dribbling balls down a zigzag path, walking the balance beam and scrambling up ropes.

One day late in the teaching year the vice principal popped into my room after hours and closed the door.

'Is everything okay, Karen?' he asked.

John was a year or two older than me and a gentle soul. Perhaps he'd seen me hobble across the playground from the carpark that morning, or perhaps he saw that I wasn't doing a very good job of teaching PE. He said I looked like I was in a great deal of pain.

I burst into tears. My right side—where RA first struck me the day I went to the beach with my cousin—wasn't responding to my meds and I'd developed an unpredictable limp. Weeping, I told John about RA. I revealed to him that my doctor had recommended hip-replacement surgery.

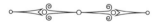

I was 28 years old. Was my job yet another thing my disease would take from me?

I loved to drive my car. My slick, red Mazda Astina was my pride and joy. To me it looked like a sports car with its pop up 'eyelashes' over the headlights. My car was a testament to how far I'd come in a little over a year. But driving it was no longer fun. It was too low for me to step into with my hip and I'd have to constantly juggle my weight from leg to leg when I was sitting at traffic lights because the pain was so bad.

Since my pneumonia attack, Dad had 'stepped up to the plate'. He was finally coming to terms with having a sick daughter. He flew from Melbourne to Sydney for my final consultation with the surgeon who was to perform my hip-replacement operation. Steve was there too—as usual he was my rock. By now Mum had met someone and moved to Queensland to start a new life. I understood her better these days and was happy for her. She needed a project and this time she was building a house. Real estate was the way Mum had decided she would make money.

Once again my decision about my next steps with my RA came down to 'quality of life'. A new hip meant I could live again. The irony was the high doses of cortisone had damaged my hip. It wasn't just the fault of my RA. I taught on the day I was admitted to hospital for my hip surgery. John and the principal, another kind man, allowed me to work right up until 17 November, just weeks before the end of the school year—and assured me that my job would be there for me the following year. Amy and her mum sent me off to hospital with a *World's Greatest Teacher* badge.

For the five weeks before my surgery I had traipsed up to St George Hospital every Friday to give blood. If I had to have a blood transfusion during my operation I wanted them to use my own blood. In 1992 AIDS was the number one cause of death in the US for young men and Arthur Ashe announced he had contracted the disease through a blood transfusion. The word 'epidemic' was all around the globe and I didn't want to take any risks.

The process of giving my own blood for a possible transfusion was uncomplicated, but it heightened my anxieties. Each time I gave blood I imagined the worst scenarios. Most of the time I imagined not waking up after the operation and how my family would react. I wasn't really scared of the pain; I was just scared about not getting through the operation. I realise now that the stress of anticipation was in some ways harder than the operation itself.

I arrived at the hospital and checked myself in. Mum and Dad were still on their way from interstate and Steve was on an overseas trip. Paul came after work. In some ways my disease had made me more introverted. More than ever, I understood that ultimately I was in this on my own. When I walked into my hospital room I felt lonely and disappointed. The room was so old and clinical. Everything was aged and yellowing. The rims of the solitary cabinet and the edges of the drapes were stained.

I knew that I had set myself up for these feelings of loneliness and distress by choosing to admit myself alone. But I was also groping to find a meaning to it all. Being alone forced me to think—whether I liked it or not. I also preferred to handle things without help, rather than burden my family or friends. Vanity came into it as well. I was embarrassed about people seeing me limp like an old, bent-over woman. I was especially guarded about letting Paul see me like this. I thought it would turn him off. Paul was doing the bare minimum for me anyway; the last thing I wanted to do was ask him for help.

Since we had separated Paul had lived right around the corner from the football club so I didn't know what he was doing most of the time. I did know that I still cared about him.

I didn't sleep much the night before my surgery but fell into a heavy slumber before dawn. The rumbling of the breakfast trolleys awoke me. My family arrived to see me before the operation—I wasn't scheduled to be 'done' until after midday. There was plenty of time for the anxiety to build up inside me. I stared at the clock for hours listening for footsteps. Finally, they stopped outside my door. The nurses came and dressed me in a blue operating gown. Underneath the gown my right leg was yellow from the Betadine which had been used to disinfect the skin. They unlocked the brakes on the bed and rolled me away to theatre. I kissed Mum, Dad, Steve and Trudy goodbye. I was in this on my own.

There are no faces I can describe, no one person I can remember. I guess that's because of the 'pre-med'. I was placed in the waiting room with all the other patients waiting for their turn to go under the knife. I had 40 long minutes to study a small whiteboard in the distance. The operating schedule was scribbled in with a black marker pen. I saw my name. Now I was scared. I took one last look at my scar-free leg and hoped that I'd made the right decision.

I was wheeled into the theatre and transferred on to the operating table. A busy energy filled the room. I looked around and saw a sea of people with masked faces, sterile gloves and blue scrubs. A triangular shape hung from the ceiling. It housed three circular lights which blinded me.

'Karen, would you like to have spinal anaesthesia only?'

'No, I want a general.'

'Karen, do you have your hip X-rays?'

'No, I do not.'

My last thought as they positioned the oxygen mask on my face was that one leg was going to end up shorter than the other because of the missing X-rays. The operation must have lasted a few hours. As I woke I wanted to spit out the foul taste of chemicals that scorched my mouth. I began vomiting and couldn't stop. The motion exhausted me. The first person I remember in the recovery ward was a compassionate, middle-aged nurse stroking my forehead,

'You made it through the operation, Karen. You'll see that the human body is amazing; you'll start to heal straight away. Can you wiggle your toes?'

I could. So far, the pain from my hip was okay. My family were there waiting when I woke up. Paul was not. I kept throwing up until Mum left. When they were gone I understood that family were the best visitors of all. They didn't require anything of me. They were just there at the end of the bed and no words had to be spoken. Dad was the best at that. He was always happy to just sit. And I liked his presence in the room. Once he was over his initial shock of seeing his daughter suffer, his energy was calming. I was glad Dad was back in my life.

As the days after my hip replacement passed I realised that Mum had a very different role. She nurtured me and rubbed my feet and shoulders hour after hour. As weak as I felt I again began to appreciate that my disease had brought us together as a family. My physical pain had somehow bonded us.

A few days later my doctor removed the pethadine, saline and drainage tubes and told me to get up and walk. It was good to be free of the IV pole, but I knew I wasn't ready. I sat upright in my bed and began to feel dizzy. A voice in my head told me 'just be stronger, just be stronger'. I tried to walk a step or two—telling myself it would show the nurses that I was strong. A loud gushing sound rushed into my ears. I couldn't resist the pain anymore. I fainted.

I don't remember being put back into my bed—but I do remember wanting my mum to stroke me and make me feel better, just like she did when I was a little girl. A blood transfusion followed a day later and I immediately felt better. However, as we approached the end of 1992 I felt I was not yet out of the woods.

> *24 November:* It's Tuesday, the weekend was lonely and I don't feel great. It is six days since my 'op'. The pain is really bad now. I am starting to become anxious about whether I can get through this. It's harder than I thought. The ward is like a 'nut house' when I sleep. There's people desperately yelling 'nurse, nurse' in the middle of the night. Distress is all around me. I am haunted by the face and footsteps of the night nurse wandering around like a stalker with her flashlight.

The nurses came in early to 'roll' me. I had to be rolled regularly in bed so the muscles around my titanium hip could begin to work. Although this was painful, it was a good thing because my bottom was killing me and I had bed sores—a by-product of the heavily starched sheets. When the nurses came to dress my wound I saw the scar from the incision and I cried. Was that vanity? It was messy, bulbous, already keloid and 22 centimetres (9 inches) long. *It felt ugly and it looked ugly. I felt ugly.* I was appalled at the sight of my own stick-thin, scarred leg. Would this scar now define me? How would my boyfriend handle the sight of it? I allowed myself to wallow in self-pity for a few days and then started accepting visitors.

Flowers, fruit baskets and cards filled my room. The phone didn't stop. I found the constant stream of visitors exhausting. I was getting bored—telling my own story over and over again. I even started to wonder whether I had concocted the story as some perverse way of getting attention. If that was the reason, I had succeeded.

Lying in my hospital bed one afternoon I saw a bunch of red, orange, yellow and blue balloons pop around the corner, then there was a sign saying 'Get well, Miss Ager'. Amy burst into my room and squeezed me tightly. It was just like our morning greetings in Grade One. Seeing Amy reminded me I'd be okay, that this would pass. She always made things better. Colleen and Amy visited many times.

29 November: Lonely day. Sundays are the loneliest and the longest. The nurses who've become my 'Monday to Friday friends' do not do the weekend shift. I had less visitors today, while all the other patients seemed to have lots. I took out my frustrations about my pain—and the absence of Paul— on Steve. I am sorry Steve. My muscles feel sore and I feel tired, but I progressed to a 'sort of a walk' on the frame yesterday. I had to carefully navigate each movement out of the room and into the corridor. It was a major accomplishment. Maybe that's why I am so tired and sore today?

I checked out my scar again and the sight of it made me cry. I am wondering why the sight of it bothers me so much. I think it's because I know what Paul will think. He'll hate it.

My day ended with a huge surprise. Lisa flew in from LA and stunned me when she walked in my hospital room. She made everything better. I love you, Lisa. What a friend!

There had been friction between Mum and me for a lot of my two-week hospital stay. We had been arguing a great deal. I felt I was a burden to her yet again and that it was my fault that her life was on temporary hold. Once more I felt responsible for her unhappiness. My blind faith in Paul didn't help.

It was that time of the year again. Paul was anticipating summer in Sydney and gearing up to party. He loved to drive my new Astina. Music pumped through the speakers in my red sports car as he flew alongside Botany Bay. I was more than happy for him to be zipping around the city in my new car, but Mum was not. She kept arguing her point.

'Why should your father and I be catching the train to and from the hospital when your boyfriend has a work van and is just using your car to run around town? And why does he have your ATM bankcard?'

I didn't want to listen. I felt she was creating this chaos, not him. Dad said nothing. I couldn't believe Mum wanted to argue with me while I was lying in a hospital bed. Mum and I clashed like opposing football teams, only Mum wasn't the opposition. Little did I know what lay ahead of me and that Mum's instincts were right.

Paul returned my car with a scratch along one side. My ATM card had been used in the city to make numerous withdrawals on nights out with the boys. I still refused to listen and again let my fears and my disease affect my ability to make healthy decisions.

I stayed longer in hospital than most hip-replacement patients. My fainting spell had scared me and it took a while for my confidence to return. Day by day I gained more strength and my passivity was slowly replaced with resilience. I began to set small goals on my daily walks. I was told that I could be discharged from hospital only when I could prove to the nurses that I could go up and down stairs with my crutches. Two weeks after surgery I finally passed the test.

Mum and Dad picked me up from the hospital and took me to my new 'home'—Jack's place—to recover. Though he was on a trip away, he'd made all the arrangements to make me feel welcome. He'd drilled holes in the ceiling for hooks and attached a rope so I could place my leg in a noose and exercise my hip. He had rearranged his bathroom so I wouldn't have to step over the bath, by attaching a long hose so I could simply stand on the bathroom tiles and wash. He was a true friend and gave my family the peace of mind they needed to leave and get back to their lives, while providing me with the luxury of feeling like I'd come home. Jack's house was exactly where I needed to be.

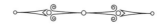

It was my first Friday out of hospital. Lisa was now back in LA. Mum and Dad had flown home after asking Paul to promise that he would be there to look after me.

My father said to him: 'If you can't take on this responsibility that's fine; but you need to tell us. If you can't then I'll stay.'

Paul promised my father he'd be there for me. A few hours after Dad left, Paul called. He was slurring his words as he said: 'You know what, I won't be coming over tonight. In fact I won't be coming over tomorrow, or the next day or any time soon. It's so over and I want out!'

I put the telephone down and I fell against the wall. I felt numb. I dragged myself into the bedroom leaning on my crutches and lay on the bed sobbing. Loneliness had not felt like this before. I desperately wanted to pick up the phone and beg him to come over, but I resisted the urge. I desperately wanted him to call back—but the phone did not ring.

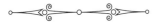

The long year that was 1992 finally drew to a close. It had started in hospital with pneumonia and ended with a hip replacement and a broken engagement. Amy's bright eyes and smile flashed into my mind from time to time. I took strength from that for a while, but it faded when I discovered my pain was deep within my heart. It was time for me to let go of my dreams with Paul and face my new reality.

I returned to St Luke's in February, the start of the new school year, with my titanium hip. The kids thought that was pretty cool.

'Miss Ager's hip is made of the stuff they put in the space shuttle!'

Life went on as normal and I continued to be separated from Paul; that is until I heard a knock on my window one night a few months into the new year.

'Kaz, Kaz.'

Sure enough it was Paul. I opened the door and with that gesture I let him back into my life—and set myself up to be mistreated once again. Before I knew it he was at Jack's house all the time. There was no sense of responsibility. He was an addicted gambler and I was fuelling his bad habits.

Chapter 7
Slipping Through My Fingers

By April 1993 I had completely recuperated from my hip-replacement surgery so I moved out of Jack's house and into my own space. My new place had views of the Georges River and was flanked by the Australian bush, just like the Lugarno house had been. I lived on the top floor of a house surrounded by trees and wildlife. I loved it. Soon enough Paul started staying over regularly and we were well and truly involved again. I had set my heart on making things work. He agreed to make a plan to save and to let me help him. Things were looking brighter.

Paul was still erratic even though there were flashes of optimism. I knew to expect his extreme highs and lows and I had learned enough to stop blaming myself for his moods. I tried to distance myself from my emotional ties to him when his temper flared. I tried to observe his moods so that 'we could get better'. I began to notice that just after Paul got paid for his week's work he became even moodier; even more unreliable.

One Thursday I decided to visit the pubs in the area. I didn't need to be much of a detective anymore. I found him at the pub around the corner from his family home. When I walked into the dark and dingy bar I found Paul slumped, once again, on a tall barstool, one foot nervously flapping along the rod that runs across the stool's width and the other foot resting sloppily on the floor. His thongs (flip flops) were half kicked aside. I figured that this was now his Thursday night venue. I felt sad to see him mindlessly tapping on the buttons of the poker machine waiting for the jackpot to show up. I wondered how often he came here and for how long. Did he just play these games after work on a Thursday or was it more than that?

When Paul looked up and saw me standing in front of him he seemed in a trance. There was barely a reaction. He just wanted to get on with the game. Winning or losing constantly dictated his moods. I started to dread Thursday nights. If he'd lost money at the pub there would be 'no weekend'. We would stay home and do nothing. This roller-coaster of emotions went on for a few months until I finally stopped avoiding a conflict and confronted him.

'You come home happy some Thursdays after you've been paid and buzzing about the weekend and other times you won't even speak to me. What's going on?'

'It's not that I don't like coming home. It's about me. When I get paid I gamble. So when I win on a Thursday I'm happy and when I don't, I get frustrated at myself then mad at you.'

I felt relief at being told this.

'I always thought it was me, but I never knew what I could have done wrong from Thursday morning to Thursday night.' I went on to tell Paul that I thought we could work together to solve his problems.

Playing card games on a machine was not, to me, 'real gambling' and I certainly didn't think about it as an addiction. Paul's admission that he had a problem made me swing into action. Immediately I slipped into my 'Ms Fix-it' role. I didn't stop to think for a minute that I had become just like my mum. I didn't want to live with Paul's mood swings, but I didn't want to live without him, either. I knew that from our time apart.

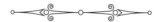

I had been introduced to Gamblers Anonymous (GA) through a guy who was going out with one of my girlfriends. He attended meetings so that he could help his brother who was battling an addiction.

'GA grew out of the pain and misery of two men, both committed gamblers, who decided they needed to change their lives,' he told me.

'They worked out the way to do it was through group meetings similar to Alcoholics Anonymous.'

It sounded good to me so I broached the subject with Paul and he agreed to give it a try. He started going to weekly GA meetings. I went to GA Partners who met across the hall. It was winter and the old church hall was damp and cold. The rickety wooden chairs felt like they would collapse under me and I often wondered what the hell I was doing there. The piercing eyes of the partners told many painful stories of homes lost, wasted years and broken families. I could see and feel their pain.

Signs saying 'One Day at a Time' were hanging on the walls. I didn't understand their meaning. I didn't appreciate that gambling is a sickness just like RA; that there is no cure, just like RA and that the addiction is predictably unpredictable, just like RA. Each day you get through is a step towards regaining control, but there's always the chance you'll get 'sick again'—just like RA. It's progressive, just like RA. I didn't stop to think for a moment that 'One Day at a Time' could have been a message for me too. At the GA meetings I also looked around with judgmental eyes and decided that Paul and I were different from these people. I convinced myself that this was just a tough patch and with my help he would get through it and we'd be out of here.

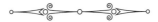

Paul had not gambled for three months when he asked me to marry him again. I accepted. I loved him dearly. I began to plan our wedding at the Sydney Opera House—the best reception venue in Australia—and paid for the photographer. We were planning to be married in nine months time, on 11 June 1994.

As the weeks and months went by I had a better understanding of Paul's problem and he became more comfortable with the knowledge that I accepted him despite his condition—just as he accepted me, RA and all.

But there was an unforeseen hurdle waiting to trip me up. Now that he acknowledged his 'disease' he could use it as an excuse. It turned out to be his best excuse.

'You don't really understand the illness—if you did you would know to leave me alone.'

I wanted to understand and I wanted to help. So I tried harder. I thought if 'space' is what he needed I would give it to him. And so I set myself up for lonely days and nights. When he said he was at his parents' home I believed him. I hung in there, ever optimistic.

Going to GA meetings started to become a contentious issue. Paul told me he wanted to take a break from them. I kept going. My world started to look topsy-turvy. He had the problem but I was getting the help. Arguments sprang up and we seemed to be fighting constantly. It was time for me to take a long hard look at every dimension of my life.

I turned again to my journal, which I kept intermittently, but particularly when I was in turmoil. Every aspect of my life needed to be balanced if I were to remain well. Keeping my journal helped me to appreciate that I was spending far too much energy on my relationship and that I was neglecting other areas like my own health and spirituality. I set the goal of finding inner peace with my health and myself. I knew that this would be a great challenge, but I knew I had to do it. I wasn't happy. I knew I didn't want to walk down the aisle into Paul's arms feeling like this so I broke off the engagement. Our second attempt at marriage had failed. As 1994 ambled on, once again we tried to sort out our problems.

4 June: I am 30 today—a momentous time in any girl's life. It has suddenly struck me that I am not going to be married. Oh God! I can't believe what a mess this is. I was supposed to be on my Hen's Night tonight and married on 11 June. Now I don't even know if I have a man worth hurting over. My 30th birthday party was karaoke. Paul got up and sang me a love song with his beautiful voice and handsome face and announced to the entire restaurant how much he loved me. This makes no sense at all. Why can't he just stop gambling? The pain of loving an addict is so great. It makes me feel alone and empty because I know I can't beat it for him. If there was another woman it would almost be easier. I am losing Paul to himself.

31 August: Things are still uneasy between us. It's always a drama when I bring up money.

1 September: Still not communicating, am facing the 'back in bed' scenario. He's not happy, but won't talk, I am managing the money, maybe that's why. He hasn't been to a GA meeting in weeks. Paul didn't buy his mum a birthday present or even a card. Selfish! But then I'm still waiting for mine and I turned 30 in June. I haven't said what I think about this, but I do feel disappointed for her. I guess it's not my business.

10 September: I can sense Paul is 'jittery'. I feel he is going to gamble. I am always worried about that now.

16 September: What a nightmare! We went to a wedding. We arrived home about 1.00 a.m. Paul rang his friend and decided to go to his mate's house (or so he said). I'm still awake at 5 a.m. waiting for him to come home, watching for glimpses of headlights down the drive. I feel nerves in the pit of my stomach, my heart is beating so fast. My body is starting to react to all this stress. I have a thumping headache. I am worried he is out gambling because he has just been paid. I keep listening for sounds of cars in the driveway.

18 September: It is 9.00 a.m., Sunday night and Paul is still not home from Friday. I am crying as I write this. I can't eat. I can hardly breathe. I feel that my disease is at war in my body. My disease is protesting against this stress. My hands, my feet, my knees, my shoulders are locked. The pain is so bad I can barely get out of bed. I know this flare is because of Paul. Tonight is the third night he hasn't come home. Three days and three nights, I just know he must be gambling again because when he is gambling I know he doesn't care about time. He doesn't care about anything when he is in that 'zone'. I am sure he has 'fallen off the wagon'.

19 September: I arrived home from school to find Paul lying on the couch. He had been unable to go to work because he was too tired and hung-over. I am so angry with him.

I am searching for answers about why he disappeared. He can offer me none. I am wondering 'did I do something on Friday night at the wedding to cause him to leave? Why did he choose now to binge?' His whole state of mind seemed to be influenced by the phone call to his mate. He must have made a plan on the phone to go to the races then. His friends just don't get that he is an addict; a compulsive gambler. I am beginning to understand that gambling is his first love, that I will never win this battle and that he will even create arguments so he can leave and be free to gamble.

I need to confront him.

'Why did you leave the wedding and go to your mates?'

'You were dancing like a wet fish, Karen, plus I wanted to see my mate. Just get off my back. It's no wonder you got bashed by your ex.'

With that painful statement I went to the bedroom and lay on my bed.

A few hours later Paul came in hanging his head and looking guilty.

'I'm sorry,' he said, crying and staring at the floor.

In that moment he won my sympathy back, but I knew I needed to toughen up. I've learned that much from GA. Tough love meant no more money from me. I had to stop feeding his addiction by bailing him out when he had no money. I also knew I needed to think about asking him to move out.

8 October: When I woke this morning I was so sore—my hands, my knees, my shoulders...it has got to be stress. I can see that Paul moving out will be the best solution to our continual disagreements. I think it's a good idea. For the first time in five years I am being strong with him. I've packed his things and am waiting for him to come home. I know I must do this.

9 October: Shit! Only one night later and Paul is staying over. Nothing has changed. The cycle continues! You idiot, Karen, what are you thinking? He came over to visit me and was all upset because he was fired for going missing during the work day. When his boss found him he was at the pub gambling so he got sacked. He turned on the tears with me, I felt sorry for him again and the cycle continues! I have to stop enabling him. It is just so hard because I love him.

23 October: I am having a really bad flare. The fingers in my right hand are really sore—so sore I can hardly write. Somehow Paul has turned his luck around. He got a new job straight away working for a friend's company in sales. But a strange thing happened today. I saw his bank balance and he seems to have too much money. He says he has been saving the last two weeks and that getting fired has forced him to change. I think I believe him.

25 October: Steve and Trudy are now proud parents and I am an aunty to Miles. Steve gets his four stripes in January. Life is better.

Early in November I had a call from the bank. Paul wasn't saving at all. He'd secured a loan for $5000 for 'our wedding'. It was all a lie. He hadn't said one word about it to me. He told me he was on the Gold Coast for his new job so when he called I asked about it and he admitted he had a loan. But he sounded terrible.

'Karen, I just lost it all at the Casino.'

'It's over, Paul, it's really over.'

I hung up the phone devastated yet again. But I knew this time there was nothing I could do to help. He was beyond helping.

Paul returned from that trip and picked up his things from my house. I still loved him, but I had to say goodbye to him—for good. I wrote him a letter:

Paul, as time passes I wonder and hope that you are okay. I wish there could have been a better way for you and for us. I know that deep in your heart you know you will have to face your demons one day. Don't forget to pray, Paul, for I truly believe that this will give you inner strength and peace of mind. It may be your last hope.

I never saw Paul again and I never posted the letter.

Paul had done a lot of damage. Physically and emotionally I was wrecked and my relationship with Mum had deteriorated. It had to be healed. She had seen all the events with Paul coming when I had my hip replaced but I didn't want to listen. Our healing began that summer on a sun-drenched beach in Acapulco, in southern Mexico.

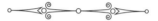

The holiday started with the simple idea that we needed to have fun together. We booked our flight and a grand resort hotel. Each day we shopped, drank wine, lay by the pool, laughed and reconnected. We sipped cocktails watching the sunset and looking out towards the Pacific Ocean and Acapulco Bay. The beauty created by the illusion that the sea, the sky and the infinity pool were one on the horizon helped to set the ambience for mending our relationship.

Breaking up with Paul had forced me to look within. Over the years I had progressed from the pain of simply getting through my days to wanting more from life. I had a better sense of self now. Walking away from Paul knowing I couldn't help him anymore, but still loving him, had forced me to challenge myself about what I wanted. I knew my life wasn't just about survival, about managing my disease and pleasing my man. Now I wanted more. One of the places I looked for that 'more' was in my relationship with Mum. We had been fighting on and off for years.

On this trip Mum shared a poem she'd written about me when my RA was relentlessly attacking.

It's my daughter, Lord, you know the one
With golden hair, who used to be such fun
Well, you've given her a cross to bear
So heavy, Lord, how is that fair?

It hurts her just to sit, nor can she barely stand
She can't get up or even raise her hand
In her eyes there is such fear
I beg you, Lord, DO YOU HEAR?

Her limbs refuse to go her way
No matter what she does, they won't obey
And now, dear God, she's blaming me
How can I handle this without some help from Thee?

I listened to Mum and tried to feel her pain and her love. I faced my fears of her abandoning us and thought about how she'd proved over and over that she would always be there for me. She had not abandoned me at all. I had judged her for leaving Dad and blamed her for my disease. I worked hard on stopping the blame game and tried to understand why she had left my father. I quit resisting that this had happened to our family and accepted her decision to go.

But I wanted to be her teacher too. I wanted her to let go of the high expectations she placed on herself to be a 'Super Mum'; to fulfill all my needs and to solve all my problems. I wanted her to think about balancing her life more evenly. She needed to stop giving up everything for me and sacrificing herself if I fell sick. And I wanted her to stop trying to control me. But what I wished for most of all was for the cycle of conflict to stop. I figured as soon as we could do this the healing could begin.

Acapulco was the beginning of our healing. We started to break down the barriers and gave each other the message that we both wanted to hear: that we loved each other unconditionally. I knew that if we could keep this up that we could have an intimate, powerful and happy mother–daughter relationship.

Leaving Paul had taken a lot of stress out of my life and, consequently, my RA was under more control. After the summer holidays I returned to St Luke's School and decided to apply for a teacher exchange program in Canada. The interview process and preparation would take the whole year, but it ended, miraculously, in success.

On Christmas Day 1995 I left for Toronto, Canada. It was yet another catalyst for change. These changes were made possible because I had reconciled with Mum and come to terms with my pain. I had stopped struggling against both.

Chapter 8
Weather With You

As I said goodbye to Mum, Steve, Trudy and my little nephew, Miles, at Sydney's Kingsford Smith Airport my inner fears about my illness flaring in a foreign country were uppermost in my mind. I knew my family was scared for me—I was scared for me too. We all silently hoped I wouldn't flare badly and end up in the hospital while I was away. We also knew that we couldn't go there in our conversations. Instead, we each filed our fears away in our minds and did not mention them.

Not facing the negative emotions that came with the disease was a defence mechanism we all used. For me, though, the emotions never went away, they just became dormant until they could manifest themselves in some other form. I boarded the silver bird, Australia's 'flying kangaroo' on a warm Christmas Day in 1995. My destination was many hours away.

I would not let my RA stop me from going on this adventure. My mindset was strong. I felt completely sure that this was the right decision for me. I was joyful despite my constant pain. My healthier attitude seemed to attract good luck right from the outset. For the first time in years I felt aligned with the universe. I just knew I had a great year ahead.

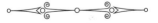

A blizzard in Toronto meant my flight from LA was cancelled. I wouldn't be tucked up in my new High Park apartment on Christmas night after all. Another delay the following morning led to an upgrade and a chance meeting on the aircraft with a 'B grade' actor. Bad weather forced us to sit on the tarmac for another hour. I noticed a passenger with two young girls—who I assumed were daughters—receiving fax after fax from the cockpit. I wanted to know why. I leant over and in a blonde moment asked: 'Are you someone famous or something? Why do you keep getting all these messages?'

'I'm the male lead in the musical *Sunset Boulevard* in Toronto tonight and I'm trying to get back for the show. It looks like they'll have to call the understudy.'

Rex Smith was handsome with a chiselled face and the aura of a star. He had been a teen idol along with David Cassidy in the United States in the 1970s. He was well known in America, but I was happy in my ignorance and had no clue as to who he was.

Rex crouched down in front of my aircraft seat and seemed keen to hear about my new adventure. As we went through Canadian Customs he handed me his phone number and said he'd show me around the city.

My new motto for the year was 'just say yes' so I accepted it.

My geographic therapy encouraged every quixotic idea I'd had about living overseas. I had an elegant home in downtown Toronto and relished my new inner-city life. Toronto reminded me of Melbourne in many ways; chic and grey with an appreciation for the arts and sport.

I was well placed by my employer who carefully matched each of the five or so teachers on exchange with an apartment and a school. I was one of the few who landed a city location. High Park reminded me of the Botanical Gardens and I lived just a few streets away from the park in an area of the same name. The suburb had a village feel about it and was urban cool. My exchange partner was gay and his place was immaculate. My home for the year was a 17th floor, one-bedroom apartment with park views. I knew I had gotten lucky.

An immediate friendship sprang up with another exchange teacher named Libby. We spent New Year together and helped each other sort out our medical cover and tax. The exchange program was brilliant because it was designed for the transition to be smooth. Our paperwork was all done and we were to be paid in Aussie dollars. We also had to sign contracts promising that we would return to our regular jobs after the exchange, but this contract proved harder to fulfill for some than others. The program took care of all other matters except for matters of the heart and losing teachers to love was common. There were many Aussie teachers who did not want to return home after their year abroad because they'd fallen in love. My new teaching assignment was a 40-minute drive from my apartment at an up-market Catholic school. My Canadian colleagues settled me in, drove me to work and helped me with my Grade Four class. Everything was perfect.

I called Rex two weeks after we'd met. He invited me to his place that night for dinner.

'I'll pick you up after I've performed the Sunday matinee.'

Rex's house was minimalist, stylish and cool. I tried not to be overawed. He was 'American intense'—but I liked the attention. He phoned two nights after our date—in between the curtain and the encore.

'I cheated and had to call you. I wanted to know if you had any comments about the other night? When can I see you again?'

It felt good for a change, but I knew I couldn't risk liking him. I didn't want my heart broken. I sensed he was capable of that. A cloudy relationship would make me tumble and fall for sure. So I focused on establishing myself in my host country and resisted his many offers to show me around the city.

I decided I needed to buy myself some transport so I went shopping for a second-hand car. I found a little Toyota Tercel, in Latin Tercel means 'one-third'—in my mind the car was three-thirds. It was a five-door manual, slightly smaller than the Corolla I had once driven at home and it ran on the smell of a oily rag. Through snowy conditions, freezing rain and flurries *Tina Tercel* got me to work and even though her column shift was on the wrong side she made my commute a breeze. I had my independence and I was ready to embrace my new city.

Rex had been calling but I hadn't seen him since our first date. A week or two later he came over and picked me up for dinner.

I wasn't used to dating. Australian men didn't date much in the 1990s, they just wanted sleeping partners; so I was impressed with the effort Rex was making. But then again it didn't take much. We had French champagne, red wine and he read me poetry. He talked about his ex-wife and cried a few tears. I got home at two o'clock in the morning—on a weeknight—but I was happy.

We started spending weekends together, shopping and sharing meals. I hid the fact that I couldn't walk well on most days. The snow helped me to keep up the pretence that I was physically fit. Everyone had to walk slowly in the snow so it became a great masquerade for my disease.

By the end of January I had progressed to the girl Rex watched television with in his sleepwear and I was the one he called to look after him when he was sick. I started staying over a few times a week. I felt unbelievably happy and that I'd finally moved on since Paul. I still couldn't believe Rex could possibly be interested in me, but he made me feel like a princess. Was this success—living abroad and dating an actor? Was he my boyfriend? I could not let these thoughts linger.

What I didn't understand at the time was how much I was allowing my sense of self to be determined by the men in my life. I had no awareness that my whole identity was being built around men, something I sensed I had learned from my mother. So long as Rex was being good to me I was happy and feeling on top of the world. My thoughts and emotional reactions to him were ruling me and defining who I was.

Life at school went on as normal, the days were long but I remained amazed at this wonderful opportunity that 1996 had brought—that I had created for myself.

2 February: A group of expat teachers travelled with me to Old Quebec City for the Ice Castle Festival. It's the biggest winter carnival in the world. Massive sculptures are carved out of blocks of ice, the weather is frigid and I am roaming around the cobblestone streets trying to speak French and drinking caribou. Caribou is a shot of brandy, vodka, sherry and port sold in the streets to warm you up. It is 25 degrees Fahrenheit—about four degrees below zero—but I haven't felt cold like I do in Sydney during winter. Sydneysiders try to 'guts the winters out' by convincing themselves it doesn't get cold there. They walk around in sloppy joes [sweaters] and thongs and prefer to wrap themselves in a rug than turn the heater on. In Old Quebec City, as in Toronto, everything is heated. There's no Arctic blast when you wake in the morning.

13 February: I called Rex. I think I was a bit demanding perhaps because I've had two weekends away and I wanted to see him. I am scared I won't hear from him again.

14 February: Rex called me for Valentine's Day and asked me to come over after the show. At 11 p.m. he cancelled. He said he was tired. Do I believe him?

16 February: I met Rex after the show for a late dinner last night. Then he called the next night and said how good it made him feel to be with me. It's nice, really nice. I think I am falling for him.

17 February: I went to see *Sunset Boulevard*. Amazing! He has quite the voice. Rex looked after me so well. I felt like a princess again. I stayed the night, the next day we had breakfast and went for a walk. I still haven't told him about my RA but I am sure he has seen me struggling. I have managed to cover up my nine inch scar from my hip replacement even though we've been intimate. I am nervous about his reaction. I am keeping the lights off.

25 February: We met for dinner and went to see *Kiss of the Spider Woman*. We went backstage afterwards and met Eartha Kitt who is famous for her role as Catwoman in *Batman* in the 60s. I had so much fun.

29 February: Rex is starting to withdraw. He says it's because it was his wedding anniversary but I am not so sure. His detachment has been without warning.

As he retreated I began to give more than I received. I had to wonder if I was setting myself up for another fall. I pursued him with phone calls—another mistake. Men are hunters, they need to chase. He finally called to tell me he was busy until the following week. It was time for a wake-up call and in my journal I gave myself a short lecture on how to behave.

> Remember Kaz take what's given and be grateful. Be appreciative for all the opportunities you've had with Rex and don't expect more. Compared to your Sydney life, this is a dream. Return to the way it was at the start of your friendship with Rex—no expectations and enjoy what you're given. Be Miss Independence and that means no questions and no demands.

Even though I was living a wonderful new life I was so far from being healed after Geoff and Paul—I still didn't grasp how profoundly wounded I had been. On the one hand I was trying to see the fullness in my life, but I also believed, deep within me, that I had nothing to give; that Rex was the one with more to offer. The pattern was familiar. I'd done the same thing with all of my relationships. Changing my geographic surroundings was never going to fix that feeling or break that pattern.

> *5 March:* It's Tuesday and I stayed over at Rex's for the second night in a row. We had so much fun. He came home after 'Sunset'. He woke me up and I got up at 11.00 p.m. We went tobogganing in the cemetery across the road. It was sprinkling snow. We played, we walked, we drank brandy and he sang. I loved it. It was living life to the fullest, being fully present and appreciating the basic things in life, like nature. Rex said it was the best time he'd had in a while. We made each other feel good. He said 'stringing two nights together back to back' was scary for him.

> *17 March*: I've been to Cancun for the spring break. Cancun was just like the Gold Coast in Queensland—slightly tacky but amusing.

I've always found Americans who travel to be a breed of their own. They're very loud, they love to drink alcohol through yard glasses and become your BFF (best friend forever) in the space of a week. Rex picked me up from the airport but he was hardly thrilled to see me. The flight was delayed and he wasn't happy. I am feeling flat.

19 March: We were supposed to go to an early dinner but he was in a bad mood so I couldn't be bothered. His personal assistant arrived this morning when I was leaving. I sense a funny vibe there.

21 March: It's Thursday night and I feel teary. Rex is beginning to remind me of Paul; his moods leave me uneasy. Poor guy though because he is a celebrity in this town there are so many people tugging him in all directions. Instincts tell me to back off, but to me Rex is Toronto; knowing him has totally changed the experiences I have had in the city. I just have to keep my 'coast along' attitude and appreciate what comes my way.

The sudden change in Rex's attitude towards me had me wondering if there was someone else in his life. Late one night, I confirmed my suspicions. I drove past Rex's house to find his ex-girlfriend's car out the front. I wasn't stalking; I just needed confirmation of my instincts so I could move on. She was also his personal assistant so they had a very close working relationship. Rex hadn't told me that they had reignited their love affair while I was away in Cancun.

I appreciated once more there was a pattern in my life of attracting men who could not love me back. I felt upset about Rex but not devastated. I felt cross with myself that I had allowed this to happen. When would I learn? I quietly blamed everything on Rex. I didn't self-evaluate at all. My association with someone famous had inflated my own ego and made me feel important. I didn't stop to think that perhaps I had long felt that the world was withholding love from me. I had felt a lack of love when Mum left, then with Geoff and again with Paul. Subconsciously, I had a feeling of not being loved enough. I had felt a lack of love in my life since I was a teenager and so I attracted little of it back.

In my mind there was always the nagging doubt that I had nothing to give a man because of my disease. I had much to learn. Chronic disease becomes a daily battle with the mind; a recurring fight to control your emotional and mental wellbeing as well as your disease. The battle never ends and it's a lonely fight.

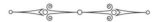

A few days after discovering the truth about Rex and his personal assistant the predictable happened—I began to flare terribly. My knee was swollen so badly that I could barely use my leg on the brake pedal in the car. It was a dangerous situation but I had to drive. I needed to get to work and I had to get to see the rheumatologist. I'd been waiting a few months until my medical cover kicked in before seeing the doctor, but now I was desperate. With my knee blown up like a balloon I knew that I needed a shot of cortisone in the joint quickly. Waiting would risk further joint damage.

I arrived at Toronto General Hospital. I lived West of Bloor Street and the hospital was North of Bloor so it wasn't too far. I sat in the car park trying to break through the pain barrier unable to bend my leg enough to get myself out of the Tercel. Eventually, I somehow found the courage I needed—that happens when you don't have a choice. Cradling my knee in the palm of my hands I pushed off with the other leg and pressed hard against the back of the seat. I had flashes of the San Souci days when Mum and Jack had helped me do the same thing.

At Toronto General I registered for my hospital card, amazed that I had access to this type of medical care in a foreign country. I limped slowly towards Room 206. The waiting room smelt musky and the magazines were well worn. A beautifully groomed lady emerged from behind Dr Jordon's dark wooden door. She had a plaster on her knee. I knew she'd had a shot. Suddenly, she fell to the floor in a fainting spell. Her husband and the doctor carefully helped her up and propped her on a seat. Watching this I began to feel sorry for myself. I knew that the doctor would inject me too but I would have to deal with the pain on my own. I didn't want to be the victim, or to tell my story to my new friends. So I kept it to myself; choosing instead to churn my story over and over in my mind, seeking sympathy and self-pity from within.

'Is someone here to drive you home?' the medical secretary asked sympathetically.

'Yes,' I lied.

Dr Jordon, an older man with a grave face but a twinkle in his eye, took a long time to examine me and then injected my knee. I'd had enough cortisone shots to understand that with a bit of pain comes the hope of quick relief. I just needed to get myself back in the car and home to bed. In the car park the attendant stared as I manipulated my body back into the driver's seat. I carefully drove myself home.

> *30 March:* I am scared. It is just two days since I have been to the doctor and I am still in pain. Pain, pain, pain! Now I have a really bad ache in my left hip and the other knee is swollen. I want to call someone, but I don't know who. I don't want to worry Mum and I don't want to be weak. Please God don't let this disease wreck my left hip too, like my right one. I am frightened and tired of this goddamn disease.

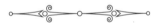

Some days I had just enough time to wash the sheets in between guests arriving from Australia. Toronto and nearby Niagara Falls were great places to show off. The Falls are simply awesome—I never tired of visiting them. In Toronto the highlights for sports-mad Aussies were the Hockey Hall of Fame, the Sky Dome and the CN Tower. The Hockey Hall of Fame is like a shrine for Canadians who are passionate about the achievements of individuals and teams who play the sport. The Canadians' love of ice hockey is like Melburnians' love of AFL. The Sky Dome (now called the Rogers Centre) was home to the Blue Jays baseball team and was famous for having the first retractable roof on a sports arena. It had also become infamous in the 90s when a sex romp by guests of its hotel was filmed live and flashed on the big screen during a Blue Jays' game. The hotel rooms had floor to ceiling windows and were the perfect backdrop for some off-field action. My Aussie visitors always found this hilarious. Another prime attraction was the CN Tower which had nothing to do with sport but intrigued everyone because it was the world's tallest building for thirty-one years. Walking on the glass floor 113 storeys high always reeled the Aussies in. When visitors arrived I usually had to increase my 'meds' and tried to block out the pain mentally.

28 April: I was reminded today of how we really have to make the most of every moment with the news that Trevor Barker, the St Kilda Australian Football legend, died of cancer. He was just 39 years old. I wish there were more I could do to impart that wisdom to the kids I teach. I feel so sad about this news.

28 May: It was Track and Field day at school today. I am wrecked from standing up all day. I hope my body can recover enough tonight so that I'll be okay to work tomorrow. I don't want the school to know I have RA. If they see me walking with a limp they're bound to ask. This illness is such a secret burden and I am so tired of it.

4 June: My family arrived from Australia to visit for a month. I've found Steve, a very pregnant Trudy, 18-month-old Miles and Mum an apartment on Yonge Street, the longest street in the world. It's so good to see them. I decided to call Rex to get them tickets to see *Sunset Boulevard*. He was obliging. This was nice as I hadn't seen him since the night I did the 'drive by' and cut my losses.

12 June: We all went to see the show and Rex really looked after us. He took us backstage and then he hosted us at his house until 3 a.m. He entertained us all. It was good to see him; he was flirtatious and holding my hand. I didn't expect this but I know I can't go there again. I have to protect my emotions.

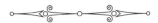

Only a few weeks later I had an unbelievable night. I saw a small advertisement in the local newspaper saying that Crowded House was playing their farewell concert at a small pub in downtown Toronto.

The Horseshoe Tavern was the place that the Australian group had found overseas success early in their music career. I couldn't buy tickets as they were sold out but I decided to try my luck at the door. I asked the bouncer if he would kindly give Nick Seymour—one of the guys in the band—a note from me, since we used to live over the road from him when I was six and he had been a good friend of my brother's. Not more than two minutes later Nick came out and beckoned for me to come in. To my surprise he remembered the Agers. He was very cool and sat there for a while before the show, telling me stories about when Mum used to drive him to primary school and how she told my brother, who was complaining about not brushing his teeth, to 'suck them clean'. This comment had stuck with Nick for years. After the gig Nick was a perfect gentleman. He sent someone to find me, took me backstage and then on to the after-show party.

I felt so privileged and sensed again that my life was really turning around for the better. My decision to leave Paul and then to move overseas had been my best and bravest move ever. Here I was in Toronto and I was on a high.

I was attracting Lady Luck.

Chapter 9
Beautiful Day

LA was the first stopover of my summer vacation. A trip to Alaska was also on the itinerary. I had worked back-to-back winters because of the northern and southern hemisphere school calendars so I was more than ready for a break.

Lisa was now married to an American casting agent, Tom—and was heavily pregnant. They lived in LA and she worked as a personal assistant to Tyne Daley of *Cagney and Lacey* fame.

I always loved seeing Lisa. She had been there for me through the hard times, we had a shared history and now her life seemed so glamorous to me. It didn't matter how much time had slipped by between visits; we fell back into our close friendship as if we had never been apart. LA had good memories for us both. We'd visited together for the first time when we were twelve. It was a dual family holiday. Along with our brothers we'd shared our first experiences of Disneyland. While Steve protected me from the battles in the *Pirates of the Caribbean* and from the steep declines on the Matterhorn roller-coaster, Lisa and I hopped aboard Peter Pan's pirate ship, flew across London in our imagination and chased Mickey Mouse around Fantasyland for a hug. Our childhood memories now bonded us.

The first few days I was in LA we hung out by the pool at *The Resort*, which was what I called Lisa's home. I marvelled at seeing my best friend seven months pregnant and secretly wished that my life would take a similar path so that our kids could grow up together just like we had done.

At Lisa's home I met Tracey—a product of second-generation, multicultural Australia—who was living in LA. Some 5 feet 10 inches tall, she had long brown hair and strong facial features. Her looks were exotic—a heady blend of Irish, Spanish and English. It was a beauty that appealed to men.

Tracey was on the 'nanny circuit' in LA. I loved hearing her stories. She was 'living in' with a wealthy, divorced American film producer whose trophy wife had 'traded up' and left him to care for his two children, a boy and a girl.

As far as nanny jobs went, Tracey had the pick of them all—a boss who adored and appreciated her, no jealous wife, two well-behaved kids, an SUV and a great place to live. I liked the sound of her life very much. Tracey and I got on well as soon as we met. She was Ms Positive and time with her and Lisa was always spent laughing about trivial nonsense. The three of us loved to indulge in Lisa's stash of Australian food. The sight of the orange and yellow Twisties (cheese twists) packet, the purple Flake chocolate bar (candy) wrapper or packets of our much-loved chocolate biscuit (cookie), Tim Tams, would send us into a chasing/feeding frenzy around the house. Lisa would ward us off, but inevitably she'd stop the tormenting and share these reminders of home with us.

As much as I missed these everyday things of Australian life, I loved everything about America in the 1990s. It was where things happened and dreams really did come true. I'd seen that with Lisa and Tracey. Everything seemed like it was 'bigger and better' in America. I didn't see vulgarity in the American culture at all and I began to yearn for a piece of it.

The Costco store appealed directly to the heart of the American psyche. At Costco's super-sized supermarkets there were low prices on every imaginable product and everything was bought in bulk. In Lisa's cupboards were not just one roll of Bounty paper towels but 15; all the Neutrogena bath products I could have wished for; the largest boxes of teabags I'd ever seen; the biggest coffee mugs in the world; three dozen cans of soft drinks and five enormous boxes of Tide washing powder. Going to Costco was an introduction to the American way of life and I found it irresistible. Having access to all this 'stuff' was a new world.

I met acclaimed actor Ron Silver on a sweltering July day. Lisa's husband, Tom—who had cast him as the male lead in the film *Skeletons*—invited me to watch the last day of filming. The Californian heat was stifling. Once you left the comfort of an air-conditioned car it was like stepping into an oven. Because of the heat I had chosen the coolest outfit I owned—a stunning, all-white sun frock which swished around my legs well below my knees. I loved this dress because it always made me feel pretty.

As the crew shot the last scenes in the film I watched from a vantage point in the fork of a huge tree—the skirt of my dress almost touching the ground.

Ron was famous for more than 80 roles in film and television. I vaguely remembered his face from the film *Reversal of Fortune* in the early 1990s and from *Chicago Hope*.

As the filming wound up I walked down a dusty unmade road and, to my surprise, Ron sauntered after me. He was a few inches shorter than me, 50 years of age and, with villainous looks and sharp features, had played many 'bad guy' roles. One couldn't say that he was a handsome man but he certainly had charisma. Or was my attraction to him more involved with my ego?

'Could you please tell me where the bathroom is?' I asked shyly.

'You can use mine in the trailer', he replied in his strong New York accent.

Expecting him to wait outside I accepted. Instead, I found myself in Ron's 'star trailer' using his toilet, while he waited patiently in his caravan-like surroundings just outside the bathroom door. I tried to tinkle quietly. My embarrassment took me away from the moment and my only thought was to escape as soon as I could.

I had no idea that he wanted to meet me and only found out later that he had asked Tom to introduce us. At his invitation I sat down at the tiny table and eyed off the surroundings. Not that fancy for a star I decided. We chatted politely for a while and he asked about my travels then astounded me with a rather special offer.

'If you would like theatre tickets any time you visit New York I'll be contactable at the Beverly Hills Hotel. Call me when you come back from your trip to Alaska.'

'That would be wonderful. Thank you,' I answered still feeling rather overawed by the turn of events.

Ron took me around the set and introduced me to Dee Wallace who I remembered from the film *ET*—she played the role of Drew Barrymore's mother.

It was 1996 and my life was changing—and rapidly. The visit to LA had been more than I could have wished for. It seemed a million light-years from the mould-infested dive of a house that I had shared with Paul in Hurstville Grove, Sydney.

13 July: Today, I arrived in Whistler, British Columbia, Canada with Libby my teacher exchange pal and her friend Emma who was also from the eastern suburbs of Sydney. Emma is tall and blonde and had overcome a fear of flying to be with us on the other side of the earth. Our spirits are high. We're staying at a homely bed and breakfast and had a great night out at the Hard Rock and Buffalo Bill's bar. We got free drinks all night because we were Aussies and things were happy, especially for Libby who was not a well little snow bunny by the end of the night.

14 July: Today was awesome. We went to the top of spectacular Blackcomb Mountain. It's the Canadian summer season and everyone was snowboarding and skiing down the slopes in blazing sunshine, wearing T-shirts! The view from the top of Blackcomb (about 7,500 ft.) of distant mountain peaks, cloudless skies and sun beams reflecting on the snow was so utterly spectacular that it made me cry. I was speechless. I think I am happiest when I am immersed in nature. I didn't care that I couldn't ski with the girls because of my RA. For the first time my mind was completely still. It was free of the usual demands I've been making on myself. I felt released. Free to truly appreciate the beauty of the moment because I was at peace within.

In the afternoon we went swimming at Lost Lake—looking up at the same snow-capped mountains that we were exploring only a few hours earlier. The 'beaches' were sandy and secluded and smelt of pine trees.

A few days later we were on the road again—three Aussie girls on a mission to drive from Vancouver to Anchorage. We had to be crazy. We continued our quest to Williams Lake, Smithers and found another gorgeous B and B which was unfortunately run by a sleazy older, single man who insisted on getting into the hot tub with me. Thinking the girls were going to join me, I agreed to a bit of heat therapy with the lake and snow-capped mountains in the background. Unfortunately the girls played a practical joke on me and went to bed. I was left, half-naked, with a stranger in the tub. The beauty and tranquillity of the surroundings were lost on me and I made a quick exit.

Libby, Emma and I were travelling around happily in our hire car until we reached the city of Whitehorse on the border between Canada and Alaska. It's the largest city in Canada's north with a population of more than 20,000. It felt more like a town to me. There we were told some bad news. Unless we paid astronomical US car insurance prices we would have to leave our hire car in Canada. Our plans were shot.

We tackled this problem in the way that many Aussies tackle many problems—we went to the pub. The locals filled us in on all the details of Whitehorse—it was 'famous' for having 19 hours of daylight in the summer; for temperatures dipping to minus 35 degrees Celsius in winter; for having the longest wooden fish ladder in the world; for Mounties and for the Klondike River Gold Rush of 1896. Whitehorse, we discovered, was not a place that inspired us to stay—even though it was also dubbed by locals as the most sophisticated city in the Territory.

Faced with the problem of getting to Anchorage without a car I was more reckless than my girlfriends. Libby and Emma took the safe option and bought bus tickets. I hitched a lift with two New Zealand guys who just happened to be in the pub having a beer too.

Looking back, I don't know why I made such a careless decision. Now and again I thought about my future with trepidation because of my RA. This fear actually became a great motivator for me at times. I truly feared becoming more disabled and not being able to live my life the way I wanted to—but during my exchange teaching year I stuck to my 'just say yes' philosophy. While this had led to many new adventures, hitching a ride with two men I didn't know was a reckless decision.

Today I would have taken note of the signs around me. When there are too many obstacles to a path of action one should back off—my inner voice was warning me. But, I didn't listen. I just waved the girls off at the bus depot and then jumped in the car with the strangers.

You could safely say my new fellow intrepid explorers were from the other side of the earth. You couldn't get much farther away from Whitehorse than the South Island of New Zealand and a place called Nelson. The Kiwi boys, Mark and Scott, loaded my baggage into their two-tone brown *Brady Bunch*-style station wagon and off we went.

A few hours into the journey I started to feel nervous, not because of the guys—they were mellow—but because of the road and the antique car in which we were travelling. The wheels were bald, the shock absorbers shot, the back of the wagon weighed down with luggage and there was no rear-vision. The trip from Whitehorse to Anchorage is 1165 km (723 miles). It promised to be a long road trip in a wreck of a vehicle with two complete strangers.

As we drove along the North Klondike Highway I had thoughts of the gold rush days when so many courageous souls braved the wilderness in search of gold and a better life. We drove about 540 km (335 miles) to Dawson City and then through the Central Yukon, catching glimpses of the Yukon River along the way.

Dawson City (which is a different place from Dawson Creek) was the hub of the Klondike Gold Rush. In just a few years its population swelled to more than 40,000 as prospectors panned for gold along the banks of the Klondike River.

For me it was intriguing to hear the local indigenous people being described as 'Aborigines'. We were still in Canada therefore they were Aborigines, not Native Americans. Now known as 'Yukon First Nations People' they gave Dawson City its culture and character. Their lives were traditionally defined by their environment—with the sun, the moon, the stars and animals forming the core of their beliefs.

Situated only 300 km (186 miles) south of the Arctic Circle, Dawson City, to me, was a strange place with locals who had strange habits. They packed the pubs at 2 a.m. in what seemed like bright midday sun and, on 21 June—the longest day of the year in the northern hemisphere—they watched as the sun set and rose again, immediately. It is one of the few cities on earth where this happens.

In Dawson City summer days are treasured—the winter is long, dark and cold. Despite the geographical differences, the place reminded me of the mining town of Kalgoorlie in Western Australia where unique characters also help define the town. If I had to describe the people of Dawson City I would say they are eclectic eccentrics. One could easily imagine the characters from *Priscilla Queen of the Desert* fronting up to do the can-can at the city's renowned Palace Theatre.

Despite all this, one day in Dawson City was enough. I took off the following day with my two Kiwi boys to cross the Yukon River by car ferry and join the Top-of-the-World Highway, bound for Anchorage, Alaska.

We were travelling on the most northern 'highway' in the world. It seemed a million miles from home. The road may have had a distinguished title but it was mostly gravel. A few minutes of it was all I needed before I began clenching my teeth and fists. There I sat for a second day, perched in between the Kiwis, my knuckles white from gripping the chocolate brown bench seat every time we shared the road with another car or diesel truck. My neck felt stiff from negotiating each bend in my mind and my eyes were pinned to the edge of the road in the hope that we wouldn't become one of the wreckages I'd seen in the canyons far below. It was a chilling drive. There were drops of thousands of feet on either side of the road and no safety fences. I kept thinking about how foolish I'd been—why hadn't I travelled by bus with the girls? One skid in the gravel would surely send us off the edge.

Finally, and against all odds, we made it to Anchorage. Despite the relief of actually getting there safely, the place was a disappointment. I met up with Libby and Emma at a youth hostel and discovered we all felt the same. As glamorous as it sounded, Anchorage was just another city. On the trip from Vancouver we had travelled through areas of wilderness and we had fallen in love with it. We all wanted to escape Anchorage as soon as we could.

The best we could do to shorten our stay was to take a quick side trip the following day. We journeyed two hours south of Anchorage to Seward, a scenic fishing town on the Gulf of Alaska. Snowcapped mountain ranges formed a sweeping backdrop behind Seward's Resurrection Bay, which was dotted with boats on fishing charters. The place was dominated by nature and the beauty was breathtaking.

The only way out for us was to go back to Whitehorse to pick up our hire car so Libby, Emma and I boarded a mini bus for the 22-hour journey on the dreaded Top-of-the-World Highway. We had no idea we would have one driver for the entire trip. He loaded himself up on Red Bull, a highly caffeinated energy drink, and drove like a maniac. To our amazement we each arrived in one piece.

Once we picked up the hire car, the small city of Skagway, Alaska couldn't come fast enough. There we loaded our car on the ferry bound for Prince Rupert, Canada, with overnight stops in Juneau and Ketchikan. On the ferry we travelled in style for a change and upgraded ourselves to a stateroom.

Our introduction to Canada's Inside Passage was awesome. Massive glacier fields, fjords, mountains and water with superb hues surrounded us as we travelled north. Juneau is a rare city in that it is only accessible by sea or air. It snuggles between towering mountain peaks that face the Gastineau Channel with a majestic beauty that left us speechless.

Next it was on to Ketchikan. Our day on the boat was punctuated by a trip to meet the ferry captain—something that had echoes of a family joke because of Mum. To be invited to the 'Captain's Table' was the greatest expression of flattery and honour to her. We decided this was a feeling exclusive to former air hostesses.

In Ketchikan we were quickly reminded that there are proportionally more males than females in this town and many, many unmarried people. Emma, Libby and I were hugely popular and we loved every minute of it. They say the only thing to do in

Ketchikan is fish or drink. We did both. We were wined and dined by Bernie, 'Dancin Dave' and other members of the US Coastguard and taken to the Coastguard Bar before a kind of sad goodbye.

We got to Prince Rupert and eventually made it back to Vancouver and, before I knew it, I was LA bound again and excited at the prospect of being with Lisa.

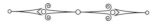

Within a day of my return to LA I was on a date with Ron Silver. I drove into valet parking at the Beverly Hills Hotel (BHH) in Lisa's BMW and gave the attendant the actor's name. It worked like magic and immediately I was treated like a VIP. I stepped out of the car and walked the red carpet to the front desk where a receptionist called Ron to announce my arrival.

Expecting to be taken out to dinner, I was surprised when Ron called room service. From that moment things started to unravel—I knew, eventually, I'd have to kiss him. This was difficult as I wasn't the least bit attracted to him sexually. However, I overcame all that and we kissed on the couch a few times and then he made his way to the four-poster bed. He sprawled over the covers, beckoning me, tapping the bed and smoothing out the wrinkles with his hand. I thought it would be childish to refuse so I moved over and perched nervously on the edge of the bed. He slid over to be closer to me. We kissed again. I wasn't relaxed. I didn't want things to get out of control. I stood up to leave. He tapped the crushed covers with his left hand and asked me to stay. He began to suck my toes. It tickled. I couldn't stop the laughter. The whole scene was surreal—I felt like an actress in a movie.

A short time later there was an invitation to stay the night. I knew I didn't want to do that. I was always so cautious. I annoyed myself in many ways and wished that sometimes I could just throw caution to the wind. My inner voice reminded me that I had just done that with Rex and it hadn't gotten me anywhere. Ron acquiesced to my lack of romance but suggested a date the following night. I lied and said I was busy. I couldn't deal with 'night time' again.

Before I left the hotel he'd asked me to the set of *Chicago Hope* where he was filming. He also offered me his apartment in Manhattan if ever I visited New York. After the rebuff I had delivered, his generosity was a shock. I left the hotel with my head spinning. Just like Rex, I wondered what he could see in a naive Australian schoolteacher more than 15 years his junior. I didn't feel aroused when I was kissing Ron but maybe that could change?

It didn't occur to me that these thoughts were actually all about my ego once again. Associating with Ron Silver made me feel important. Even the simple act of 'valeting' Lisa's car and saying Ron's name to the valet guy made me feel superior and special. Ego! I liked the image of Karen Ager attracting attention because of whom I knew. Ego! It made me feel powerful. Ego! I couldn't see that once again I was relying on a man to make me feel good.

The next morning Lisa and I 'glammed' up and went to the set of *Chicago Hope*. Ron was there to greet us and to show us around. We met Mark Harmon and I was made to feel very special again. I couldn't help but think here we were, two Sydney girls in Hollywood. Ego! As we left I declined an invitation for dinner that night. But two days later I was on another date with Ron at the BHH. This time it was lunch. Perhaps Ron thought he was getting 'lunch with sex on the menu'. This time kissing him was very nice.

That night he invited me stay for dinner and to a party on Sunset Boulevard with his manager. He said he'd be proud to take me and that there would be a lot of stars there. I didn't care and declined. I didn't want to lead him along. Our brief 'friendship' was sure to be over since I had squashed all his advances like floating bubbles in the air. I thought there was no way he'd pursue me because I hadn't allowed him to move past kissing me. I understood later that I had grossly underestimated him and that I hadn't counted on Ron's integrity as a man.

Again I was swinging between feelings of adequacy and inadequacy.

4 August: Lisa and I had laughing fits twice today. We just could not stop. To me this is a rare and wonderful happening that only occurs between friends who have a shared history. We didn't even know what we were laughing about.

5 August: I went to the obstetrician with Lisa today. The baby is due in about a month. When I saw the heart beat of her child on the ultrasound I cried. I couldn't believe that we were now so grown up that she was about to be a mother. I wished with all my heart that I was pregnant too.

Rex called out of the blue today. He told me his stage show, the musical *Sunset Boulevard* was moving from Toronto. He said he hoped he could see me when I returned to begin the new school year. He asked if he could stay two nights once his house was packed up. I didn't know I was his best friend.

14 August: Austin Ager was born today. He was six pounds nine ounces. I can't believe Steve and Trudy had another boy. I thought Trudy was having a girl for sure. I haven't spoken to Steve or Mum yet. I am a little upset I am not there to share the joy.

When I am talking about my father's eccentricities I tend to call him Max. This is 'classic Max.' He called the hospital to check on Trudy and somehow got put through to the delivery room telephone right when Trudy was in the middle of giving birth. Typical Max!

17 August: I have arrived in Philadelphia. I am visiting 'friends of friends'. I don't really know them. They are taking me to the Jersey Shore, a strip of continuous beaches and seaside towns on the Atlantic coast. I already feel worried about not being able to walk fast enough to keep up with the group because of my RA and about explaining my scar on the beach. I am also starting to get concerned about money. The summer is coming to an end and I need to get home to Toronto and pay my bills. I think I'll be home every Saturday night for a month. That wouldn't be a bad thing! I also need to see my doctor. I don't feel great.

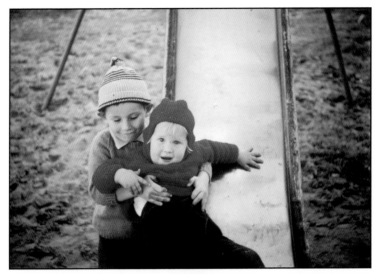

Home to Australia from Lae, Papua New Guinea in 1965. My brother, Steve, and I play on the slide. He's ready to catch me if I fall. I would come to understand that he would never waver in this resolve.

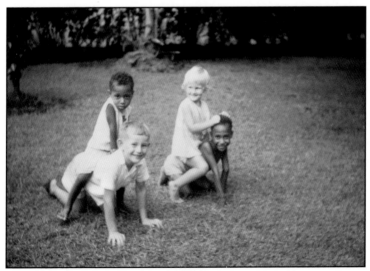

Steve and I playing with our friends in the backyard in Lae, Papua New Guinea in 1966—I sobbed when I left my friend Martarema behind when we returned to live in Australia.

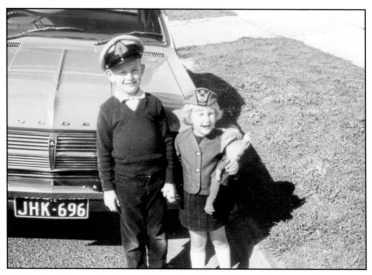

My brother, Steve, and I pretending to be airline cabin crew in front of the family's Holden car. At 6 years of age, Steve knew he wanted to fly aeroplanes—1968.

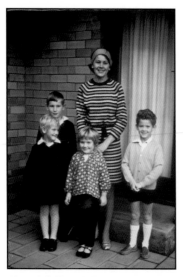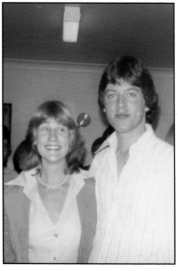

Above left: Friends for life. At home in Lower Templestowe, Melbourne— anticlockwise is Mum, Steve, me, Lisa and her brother Mark. Lisa is looking characteristically mischievous—1970s.

Above right: My cousin David and I just months before my first attack on the beach—late 1970s.

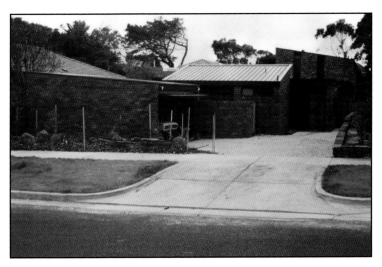

Perfect from the outside looking in: my parents' Black Rock dream 'home'. It was built so Steve and I could have fun. Now I know how hard this is to achieve and how easy it is to lose—1975.

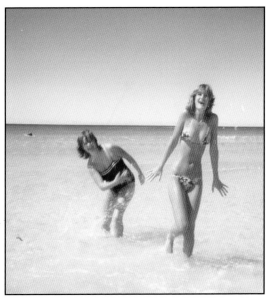

RA free. Me being splashed by one of my high school friends at Black Rock Beach. The beach and water have always been a special place of retreat for me.

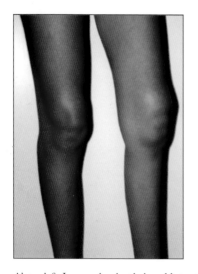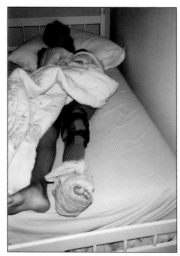

Above left: I remember just being able to stand unaided for this photo. My rheumatoid arthritis attacks my knees and my spirit. Sans Souci, Sydney—late 1980s.

Above right: My RA attacks again. Another bitter assault. This time I am bedridden. Mum and I resort to bandages and then scarves to help support my joints. Life didn't seem worth living.

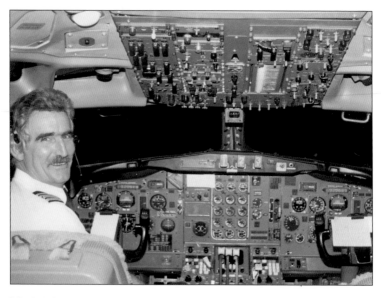

My dad, Captain Max Ager. He was passionate about flying—and still is—mid 1980s.

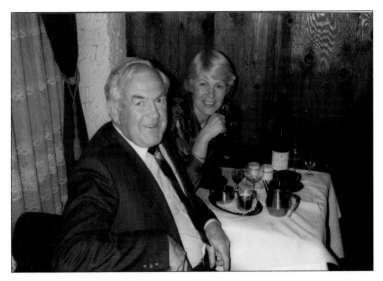

A moment of respite for uncle Jack and Mum in between carrying me down four flights of stairs for hydrotherapy treatments and feeding me—1988.

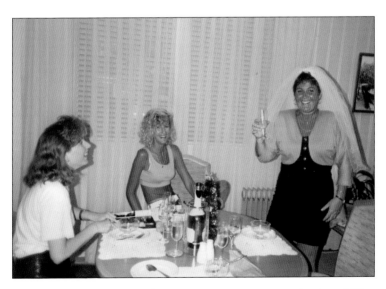

Lisa, 'The Wedding Planner', her sister-in-law and I (middle), goofing around. The smile was just a mask for my pain and my skeletal frame shows it—late 1980s.

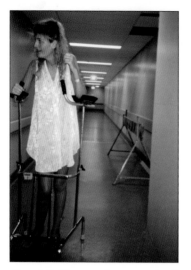
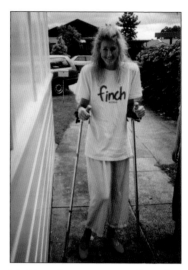

Above left: On my walker recovering from right hip replacement surgery. I wasn't allowed to leave hospital until I had conquered the stairs—1992.

Above right: Returning 'home' to uncle Jack's after my hip replacement. Still smiling—1992.

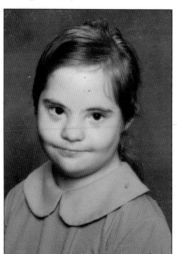
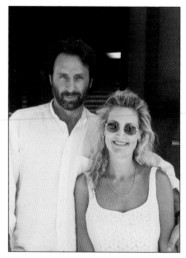

Above left: My inspiration for life, beautiful Amy. Pictured here in Grade 1. She's feeling so proud to be photographed in her school uniform; you can just see it in her eyes—1992.

Above right: Friend Ron Silver and I. He was the catalyst for my move to New York. Ron helped me to rebuild my self confidence. He was always a true gentleman to me—1996.

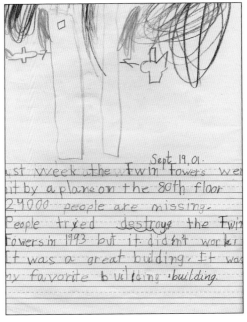

ast week the Twin Towers wer
hit by a plane on the 80th floor
24000 people are missing.
People tried destroy the Twin
Towers in 1993 but it didn't worker
It was a great building. It was
my favorite building building.

Sept. 19, 01.

September 11 through the eyes of a child. (Published with permission and courtesy of parent and child.)

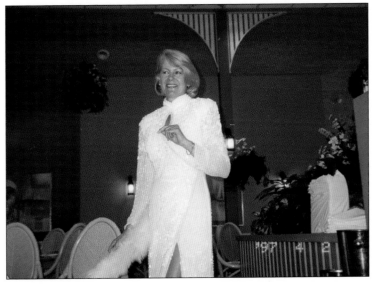

Mum was still modelling at 59; by now she'd been on the catwalk for 40 years but she was still beautiful.

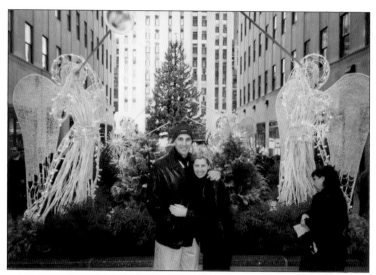

My brother, Steve, and his wife Trudy in front of the Christmas tree at the Rockefeller Centre 2001. Trudy had beaten her own health issues to be in New York. The tree lighting was a symbol of hope for a brighter future.

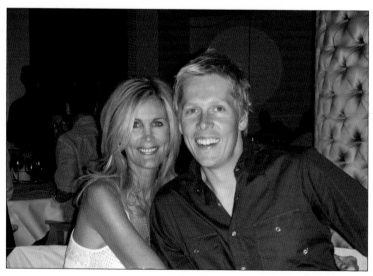

Matt and I in London, May 2006. We had just achieved Green Card status in the US and were so happy.

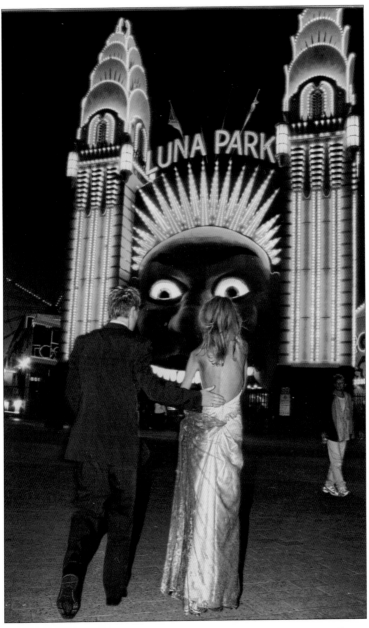

Matt and I married on 4 July 2004 in Sydney. I had finally found someone to love me unconditionally despite my RA.

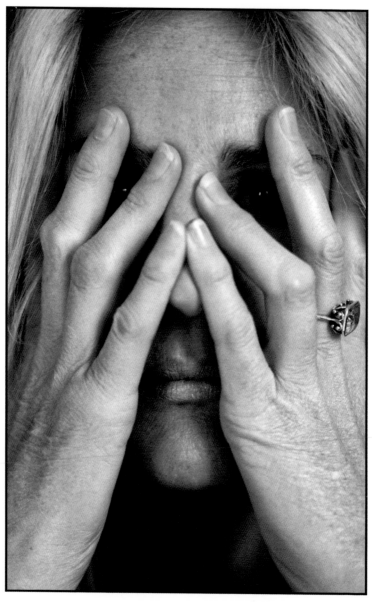

RA's betrayal can be seen in my hands. (Photo courtesy Haik Kocharian).

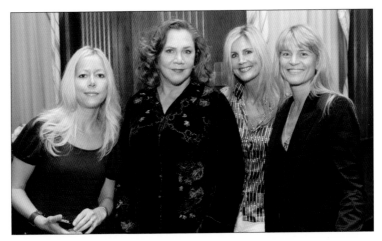

Charlotte, Kathleen Turner, me and Venessa at an Arthritis Foundation event in New York City. By this time I was sitting on the New York Chapter's board of the Arthritis Foundation and speaking on behalf of the millions of people who suffer from the disease worldwide. Ms Turner has RA too. My girlfriends are always there to lend a helping hand. (Photo courtesy Arthritis Foundation NY Chapter.)

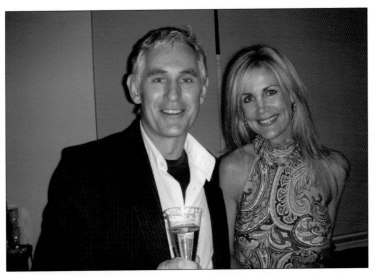

My brother, Steve, on Christmas Eve 2006. He didn't know I'd had an embryo transfer that day. I am feeling hopeful that by the new year I'll have my own bundle of joy to buy Christmas presents for.

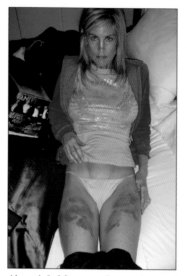
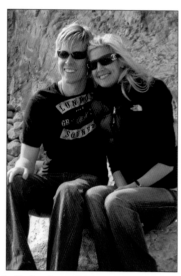

Above left: My eyes reflect my battered spirit. Bruises from IVF injections cover my legs; but I still wouldn't give up—2006/2007.

Above right: Matt and I on the beach in Malibu, California in April 2007. I was happily ignorant of what lay ahead in the coming weeks.

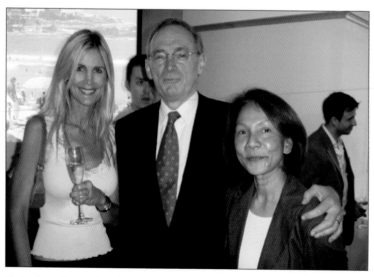

Retired premier of New South Wales, Australia's largest state, Bob Carr, his wife and I at an 'ex pat' function at the Australian Consulate in Midtown New York. I am always proud to be an Aussie in New York City.

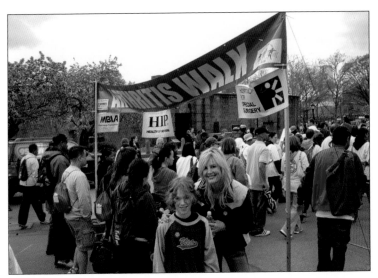

The Arthritis Walk at Battery Park, New York City in 2008. I am with Joseph Lebowitz, my past grade 2 student. He walks every year to support me. Joseph and his family have raised thousands of dollars over the years to help find a cure for arthritis. He wants his teacher to 'be well'.

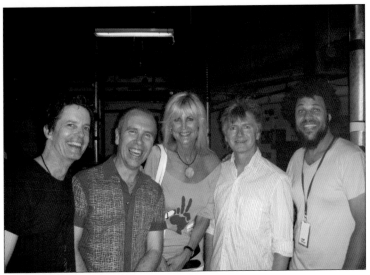

Crowded House perform in New York in 2007. I was lucky enough to get the chance to catch up with old friend Nick Seymour after the show.

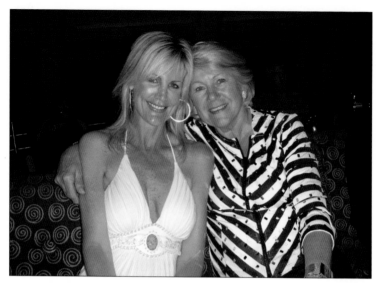

Happy with Mum celebrating her 70th on a Pacific Cruise in 2008. Dad was even there! My eyes are sad because Matt was not with us.

Little Willy, our new family member. He has brought us so much joy. Willy's love has helped me to be more peaceful about not being able to conceive a child.

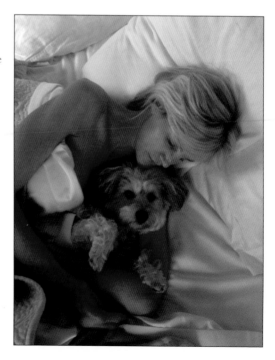

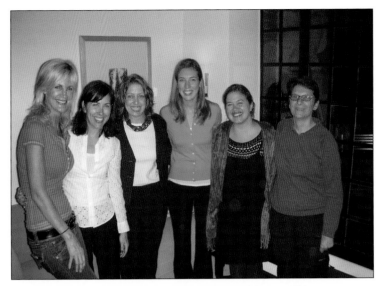

The first meeting of the Karen and Arthritis Support Group in Midtown Manhattan in 2009. The group has been growing ever since.

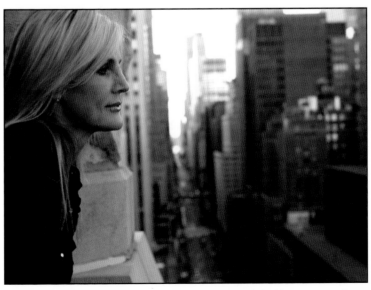

I still call Australia home but New York from our terrace is looking pretty good. (Photo courtesy Haik Kocharian.)

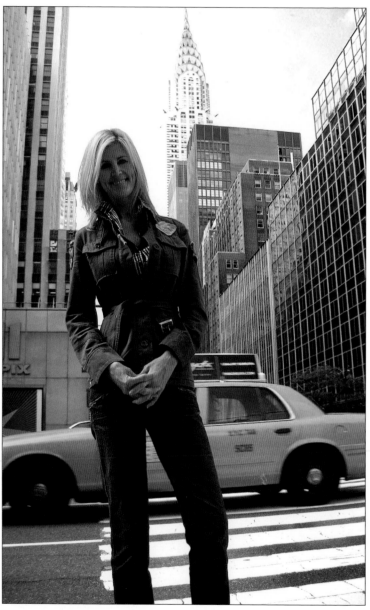

42nd Street in New York; the city I fell in love with.
(Photo courtesy Haik Kocharian.)

24 August: I took the train from Phillie to Toronto. I don't like trains much and it took about ten hours to get home. It was brutal. Rex called and wanted to take me to dinner in High Park. I rallied after the long journey and surprised myself by being well enough to go out. He picked me up and charmed me straight away by wearing a suit. He is leaving for Vancouver in a few days. He didn't need to stay with me in the end. He said he just wanted to see me. I was seduced. We had an amazing night. I ended up staying with him, we had breakfast together and went walking through the cemetery one last time and he played the guitar for me. But tonight, a day later, it's after midnight and he hasn't called like he said he would. He is so unreliable. I can't believe I was stupid enough to be seduced by him again.

25 August: Rex finally called (a day late). I was really annoyed and told him so. I let him know that I deserved better. I think as time goes by he'll feel bad about this. He needs to hurry up and leave for Vancouver now!

29 August: I went for a consultation today about my hands. They are deformed from the RA, bulbous at the second and third knuckles of my right hand. The doctor said he doesn't want to fix them at this stage. He told me the joints have fused in the 'best way possible'. The wrists and thumbs have fusions. The fingers have fused in a way that they look okay and not like claws. I think it was good news!

10 September: Lisa gave birth to a baby girl today—Meg Patricia. After 21 hours of a difficult birth the doctors were forced to do a caesarian section. I can't believe my mate is now a mum. Time for us to grow up. In just over three months I'll be homeward bound. The countdown is on.

Ron Silver called, out of the blue and invited me to go to New York. He said he would look after airfares and anything else I need. I didn't know what to do. A few nights before his call I saw him in a movie. He was kissing the actress's toes. I laughed and wondered if that's where he got the idea from when he kissed my toes at the BHH.

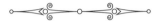

October delivered a reality check. I felt really unwell and had severe tenderness in my left hand. The pain was getting me down and I felt like I was on the slope of a steep hill and falling. The legacy of my wonderful summer holiday was a vicious RA flare. My knee was swollen yet again and was so full of fluid that walking was nearly impossible. I was so tired of fighting RA on my own.

At the Toronto General Hospital I was led by a petite woman to one of the tiny, familiar treatment rooms. Slowly I changed into a blue surgical gown, leaving the opening towards the back. Luckily I managed to wrap the tie twice around my waist so that I could fix a bow at the front to secure the garment. My arms wouldn't bend at the elbow and my wrists couldn't twist to tie it at the back. White tissue paper was scrolled along the medical table waiting for me to sit my body down—if I could. I was too sore. The metal rings made a whirring sound as the green hospital curtain was pulled closed. I felt that I was behind a barrier that separated me from healthy people on the 'other side'. The injection was prepared as I sat and waited, staring at the curtain and counting the number of silver rings. I knew that this was an attack I had to face on my own. But I was growing used to that. There was no choice in the matter. Like the soldier going to battle I had to overcome my fears. Only cowards desert.

My body was rigid as the sharp steel needle pierced my skin. I felt the cold liquid cortisone shoot into my swollen knee joint and then dissipate into my flesh. I flinched and kept my teeth clenched, my mouth tightly shut. The needle slid out and pressure was applied to the puncture wound. It was over and I would be rewarded with a brief amnesty in the fight that was taking place inside my body. The curtain was pulled back and I returned to the healthy world—until the next time.

8 October: I went to church today because I felt the need to go. When I got there I knew why. It was as though God had summoned me because it was a mass for the sick. The priest talked about how sickness is like being broken and that instead of feeling that it is the absence of God one should consider it is his presence.

I wonder.

Chapter 10
Empire State of Mind

A phone call: Ron Silver! He really wants me to visit him in New York City and called to invite me again. I still can't help but ask myself the question: 'What's he calling me for?'

Another phone call: Rex! He wants me to visit Vancouver.

'I don't want you to disappear without saying goodbye.'

My exchange year was quickly coming to an end and the friendships I had formed were beginning to take on a new energy. I liked it.

> *20 December:* I am feeling very nervous about arriving in NYC to stay with Ron. I do like him and I know that I could control things with him sexually if I need to. He has been so generous with all the arrangements. He sent me an airline ticket and his personal assistant booked my flights and our dinner reservations. It was all done for me. Ron told me to catch a cab into Manhattan from the airport, I guess that's a 'New York thing'.

There's power in New York City, you feel it as you approach the landing strip at JFK airport. Energy is in the air, even before you land. It hits you like wildfire and pumps adrenalin through your veins. There's a swirl of emotions filling the cabin; an air of excitement, anticipation and fear. I'm scared. Would this city gobble me up and spit me out? I couldn't dismiss my fears. Yet it didn't make any sense to feel so nervous. Was it New York or was it Ron that was making me anxious? I couldn't tell.

From above and to the untrained eye of a first-time visitor, the island of Manhattan looks like it's divided into two cities. The southern end of the island (I now know to be 'Downtown') was dominated at the time by the vertical impact of the Twin Towers and, further north, the denser skyline is governed by the Empire State Building. The Empire State dwarfs all other skyscrapers, while the flashing lights of Times Square, just ten blocks away, make another strong statement about the city. It's an invitation to have fun. Some force pulsates through the aircraft until touchdown as if all the thoughts of the passengers—their expectations et al—are actually generating a sort of electricity. What lies ahead for them in New York City? There's the promise of a good time and a real sense that we're about to land on, as R. Shorto described in the title of his book *The Island at the Centre of the World*.

I became an instant New Yorker the moment I arrived at JFK airport and hailed a cab for the 30-minute drive to the Big Apple. The line of taxis looked as if they were little yellow beetles crawling through the alleyways under the bark of an old groaning elm tree while inching their way slowly ahead, row by row, to who knows where on the island of Manhattan. As I drove over the Queensborough Bridge I could see Manhattan's skyline once again—this time from ground level. New York sparkled like diamonds on a tiara. She was majestic and even more beautiful than I expected. Her crown jewel: the Chrysler Building. Grand and regal in appearance, the Chrysler Building looked like she too was wearing a diadem. Art deco in design, it was developed in the early 1930s by automobile magnate W.P. Chrysler. Its spire was hoisted in just 90 minutes in a race to elevate her to win the title of Tallest Building in the World. Sadly, it was a distinction she kept for just less than a year when she was over-shadowed by the Empire State.

The Chrysler Building captured me from the moment I laid eyes on it. Graceful and elegant, yet bold in its statement about American capitalism, it gave the city even more character and formed the perfect backdrop for my stay on Park Avenue.

I arrived at Ron's upper eastside apartment in time for dinner. 'Upper eastside' was a geographic term which meant nothing to me at the time. At least the taxi driver knew where he was going, even if I didn't have a clue. The area bustled with life. The building's rather pompous doorman greeted me and said I was expected. I wondered what the doorman knew about Ron and who he thought I was. *Stories of an Upper Eastside NY Doorman*—what a great name for a book I thought, as I imagined the tales of 'Husband Huntresses' and 'Doggie Divas' that could be told.

Author Plum Sykes coined the phrase 'Husband Huntresses' about wicked New York women who only pursue other women's husbands; I bet Ron's doorman had seen a few of them visiting here, I thought. As I stood in the lobby waiting to be announced, a 'Doggie Diva' came skipping in from Park Avenue with her pet 'pooch' called Tugboat. I wondered if the pug was just a toy for flirting. It all felt so foreign to me. As I caught the elevator up to Ron's apartment I had butterflies racing around in my stomach. Ron put me at ease as soon as he opened the apartment door by taking my bags into his kid's room.

'You can sleep here if you like.'

He'd shown me his integrity yet again. There was an authenticity about Ron that I was beginning to like.

I was immediately struck by how small his NY apartment was. The Australian in me was saying 'only two bedrooms and a small, windowless kitchen'. I wasn't being *urban bourgeois* I was just used to space—Aussies are. But space is at a premium in New York. If you actually have a kitchen in Manhattan and not just a sink, bar fridge and microwave behind some pull-out doors you're doing extraordinarily well.

'It's just New York,' Ron explained as he read my mind about the size of his apartment.

'There are a lot of people, not much space and crowds wherever you go. It's a test of your patience and sometimes your senses, but the city is enchanting.'

So what was it about New York that was so captivating? My love affair with Gotham began immediately. I loved her because of her energy and I wanted to know more. Gotham, the name hip locals affectionately call the city, came from a real town in England where local villagers had the reputation of being mad. It's a buzz word for the trendsetters.

Ron began to explain a little about the city he had been raised in. I was conscious that I needed to learn as much as I could about New York if I was going to understand what made her beat. The city had a pulse and I wanted to put my finger on it. Frank Sinatra's song 'New York, New York' kept ringing in my ears. I wanted to know why it was so hard to 'make it there'. Why is it that so many people come to New York to chase their dreams? What gives the city its rhythm?

It was obvious to me from visiting Ron was that you needed to have some serious money to live in NY. But I knew that. I also knew about the *New York Times*, the NYPD and the Yankees. Everything else I knew about New York was because of *Seinfeld* and neurotic characters like the Soup Nazi and George Costanza. I understood that New York women dated a lot of men because of Elaine's character in *Seinfeld*; that apartments housed bikes and that Kramer had a penchant for bursting through Jerry's door. I didn't know if all apartment living in New York was like that—or if they met regularly at the local diner instead. This hardly made me a knowledgeable tourist. I wanted to know more about New York so that I could understand why my feelings about this city were so intense.

Ron began my orientation by introducing me to the five boroughs of New York: Manhattan, the Bronx, Queens, Brooklyn and Staten Island. He explained that Manhattan and Staten are islands; Brooklyn and Queens are situated on the western end of Long Island and the Bronx is the only borough on the US mainland.

He went on to outline the history of the city—which was originally inhabited by Native Americans who sold it for a handful of dollars' worth of glass beads. By the end of his little lecture I knew it was named 'New Amsterdam' in 1624 by the Dutch and was later taken by the English and that today the city is a melting pot of cultures, with 36 per cent of the population not born in the US. Later I was to learn where the nickname 'Big Apple' came from. Originally a racing term used by New Orleans stable hands in the 1920s, it was picked up by a newspaper writer and used in an article. New York races meant big money and for the horses this meant a bigger apple. The phrase stuck.

Ron's lounge-room was decorated in an elegant, stately manner. Hundreds of beautifully bound books filled his shelves, all standing upright as if at attention. It was a somewhat daunting sight and quite a symbol of his intellect.

We took an elevator down to a restaurant on a lower floor in the building. The maître d' was expecting us. I was too nervous to eat so I tried to focus on the conversation. Luckily Ron, apart from being a charming companion, had enjoyed a busy life and had plenty to talk about. He said that he had worked for the CIA in the 1960s on intelligence-gathering missions in Russia and Asia. I was fascinated—but totally out of my depth. I had a very limited ability to offer much in a discussion about the CIA—my knowledge was derived totally from TV and the odd spy book I had read. As well, I wasn't very globally aware. I think I'd lived in Hurstville Grove for too long.

I've since learnt the value of being a good listener. If I'd appreciated it then I might have felt more confident. Our conversation soon turned to politics—Ron supported the Democratic Party at the time and was very politically motivated. Again I felt nervous and insecure about my inability to talk to him on his level, but knew that I could develop a healthy understanding of American politics if I had to. In that moment though, I was at the dinner table and we were sharing a meal and I had little to contribute about the party the country had just voted in to oust the Republicans. I had to wonder at the time whether or not he was bored? What the hell was he doing here with me, a teacher from Down Under?

As a group, we teachers have a tendency to underestimate ourselves—we put ourselves down when we are out in the 'real world'. The truth is we are amongst the hardest workers in any community. We work countless unpaid hours of overtime, constantly multitask and our influence is huge, whether it's good or bad. Teachers do so much more than 'just teach', but because we're seen—by a few— along with dog walkers and cleaners we sometimes view ourselves in the same way. If I had I known that Ron was an ex-high school teacher and the son of a teacher, I may have had more faith in myself. I might have even been able to settle down and enjoy the evening.

By this time I was also becoming rather distracted by my own body. I wasn't feeling very well with my RA and I had stomach cramps. But there was no way I was going to mention this to Ron. We talked a while longer. I was enjoying getting to know the man and found him to be rather fascinating.

Bill Clinton was the President-elect at this time and the inauguration was coming up in January. Ron raised the subject and then said:

'Karen, I'd really like it if you would accompany me to the presidential inauguration. I have a dress for you to wear. You know about my ex, well I had bought this gorgeous gown for her but we were finished before I had a chance to give it to her. It's beautiful—if you don't mind wearing it.'

I felt completely overwhelmed by this amazing invitation. We talked dates. Working out that the date of the inauguration was after my scheduled departure date, I thanked him for the invitation but said I would have to decline. He then asked me if I could change my flight.

The reason for my lack of enthusiasm—despite the fact that half of America would give their eye teeth for such an invitation—was that I was secretly worrying about where I would sleep in Washington DC. There was no reason *not* to feel completely comfortable with Ron. He had always done what he had said he was going to do. There was no question about his morals. I just didn't trust him because I didn't know how to trust. So I told myself that if I accepted his invitation it would be assumed that I would sleep with him. '*I* wasn't like that', I thought, putting myself on some moral pedestal. I didn't want him to think that I was just like other women who would probably sleep with him to get to the inauguration. I did not understand that I was projecting the pain of my past on to him. If I had been older and more experienced my answer would have been different. I would have understood that Ron was an honorable man and I would have had the self-confidence to control the situation sexually. I misunderstood his intentions, forgetting about the power that women hold sexually. We're usually in control at least until they've slept with us and then it all changes. I was in the driver's seat but I didn't know it.

My stomach pains were getting worse—I was now convinced it was nerves. It had been a huge day.

I had completed my year of exchange the same day that I'd flown to New York to visit Ron. My emotions were shot. Before I left Toronto I'd had a day of saying goodbye to the children in my class and to my colleagues. I was leaving the kids in the middle of their school year and this made me feel guilty. Ron's kindness and invitation and all my sad farewells made me start to feel like I wasn't ready to go home to Australia.

The school year had flown by with relative ease. I'd worked hard and there had been a few challenges—but not too many. One of my students, Michael, desperately needed to be understood and was crying out for help. He'd do anything for attention, including knocking all the stacked chairs off the tables in a classroom after school was out. He was the one to whom I did not want to say goodbye—I felt I could have made a difference to his life if I had been there for the whole of the Canadian school year. And then there was Angelo whose family had been turned upside down by the birth of his Down's Syndrome brother. Angelo didn't get the attention he once had as an only child and his parents had reached out to me in a desperate search for support. I told them about Amy and we felt connected. They felt understood and, in turn, little Angelo benefitted.

I had also been caught up in strike action by the Catholic Teachers' Union. Even though I wasn't part of the union in Ontario I was expected to support it. The teachers had decided to 'work to rule' to support their case. This action meant that you could only work normal school hours. There was no working back, no taking assignments home for marking, no personal money was to be spent on rewards for the class, no after-school meetings were allowed and there was to be no report writing permitted at home. It was only then that I gained a true understanding of what we as teachers do beyond our job description. That's when I really appreciated teachers do 'more than just teach'. I hadn't stopped to think about it before.

I went for my final doctor's visit a few days before the end of school. Dr Jordon was happy with my progress and so was I. I had less painful swelling and my disease felt more under control.

The letter he gave me reported on my condition:

I saw Karen for a final visit 17 December 1996. She is making good
progress. Karen is still having some palindromic episodes (pain, swelling and
fluid retention), but her energy and sleep patterns are fine. No deterioration
in any of her joint regions except for continuing crepitus (grating) of her left
knee that has interfered with her regular swimming activities.
I had seen her earlier in the fall and injected her right knee and later on 28
October. Her right third PIP (finger joint) had joint swelling that had been
increasing in the previous 3 weeks.
On examination she looked well. Rheumatoid deformities as before. Her
regular medications include as before, Prednisone, Imuran, Caltrate,
Naproxen, folic acid and now after almost 8 months Chloroquine 250 mgs
daily.
She leaves here 23 December with expected arrival home 10 January 1997.

None of these drugs were a cure for RA—there's no such thing yet—but if I could balance the better quality of life they gave me with the inevitable side effects, then I figured I was doing well.

The trip to New York had been a 'last minute get away' because Ron had invited me. I planned to spend Christmas with my old friend Lisa, her husband Tom and baby Meg in LA and go to Vegas for the New Year. My head was spinning at the dinner table with Ron. Reality suddenly hit home. My Canadian farewells hadn't seemed real because I would see the teachers I'd been on exchange with at home in Australia. The fact was I had a night left in New York and two nights in Toronto, then my east coast adventure would be over. I wasn't sure I was ready for that. I drifted away and started thinking about my trip home to Australia in early January. The conversation with Ron wafted over me.

Going through my head was a procession of doubts, worries and fears about the future—perhaps prompted by my unexpected stomach pains or simply because a very special year in my life was coming to an end. Other expat teachers had returned home and then resigned because of love. I was not unsettled because I had fallen for a man—instead I'd fallen in love with life.

Since I had been in Canada my whole attitude had changed. My disease had slipped into remission and I was enjoying everything—for the first time I could remember. It was unbelievable to be so full of energy and totally happy and joyful about every little thing that happened, everyday. Gone were the times I spent telling myself that I'll be happy when... Instead I was enjoying each moment. The problem was I didn't know if my happiness was just due to the fact I was overseas or if it were something more. The prospect of living in the outer suburbs of Sydney just didn't excite me anymore—but I was hoping my new-found love of life would return home with me and cast a rosy glow on life in Oz. I loved and missed Australia—and my family—very much. I wondered if this would be the catalyst that would propel me further along my road to fulfillment and contentment.

The procession of thoughts that I was ploughing through as I sat at the dinner table with Ron presented another unnerving thought: RA. I brushed aside my anxieties about going home, telling myself that my illness had always been my biggest obstacle and now that I had addressed it and my RA was somewhat under control, no other obstacle would ever be as insurmountable.

But RA was only a part of my emotional landscape. Sure, it had happened to me and life had been hard because of it—but I had let my arthritis become me. I still didn't really know myself. I wasn't even 'awake' enough to acknowledge my anxiety about going home to Australia, or even allow myself to really feel my apprehension. So I shoved my fears aside, leaving them to lie dormant until I got home.

After dinner Ron and I went back to his apartment and talked some more. I stayed the night—in his kid's room. There was no pressure to sleep with him. He was a gentleman and a very gracious man and I had—and still have—the utmost respect for him. However, he was growing on me. I was becoming more open-minded about the thought of being with an older man because he was so charming and so endearing.

We talked about his rather bumpy love life—he was still recovering from a series of broken relationships and needed to talk about them. Our conversations saddened me. I listened again during breakfast at the very plush Regency Hotel on Park Avenue. He wanted to chat about his kids, his ex-wife and the glamorous anchor-woman of a television news show on the West Coast he'd been dating and rejected by. Later we enjoyed a walk through the bustling streets of New York—Ron wanted me to see the Christmas windows at Saks Fifth Avenue and the tree in the Rockefeller Center. All this effort he was making just for me. I didn't stop to think that Ron could be Jewish and didn't celebrate Christmas, but Hanukkah.

It was four days before Christmas and New York City was hectic. The crowds were dense, the sounds intense and I felt like I was being pushed along the pavement at the whim of the masses—like white-water rafting through rapids. We walked from his apartment, but I had trouble keeping up with his pace because my feet were sore. He was a local and was skillful at negotiating the currents of people and avoiding the deadwood. I knew I couldn't tell him about my RA because I believed he'd want to run; so I pretended I was okay, just a little tired. The great cover-up continued.

I was awestruck by the height and dominance of the Christmas tree at the Rockefeller Center—and dazzled by the beauty of its decorations. The lights were sprinkled all around like stars in the sky. Children were ice-skating to 'I'm Dreaming of a White Christmas'; their loving family members standing by watching and cheering them on at every completed circuit. I couldn't believe this New York moment was happening to me.

There was good energy everywhere except it bypassed Ron completely. His face was familiar to many Americans on Fifth Avenue. He started to look agitated. The crowds intensified his feelings. Suddenly he wanted to get home quickly. The attention from the public was getting on his nerves. I felt their eyes on me too. I could feel 'them' making judgements about me. I tried not to take notice of the stares. I felt proud Ron had chosen me to walk by his side through the streets of New York. I knew he had to be careful about who accompanied him in public, so I took it as a compliment.

I left NY a few hours later with the invitation to President Clinton's inauguration still open and an invitation to move into Ron's NY apartment. He said if I liked New York I could live there for as long as it took me to get established and find a job. It all sounded so exciting.

But was it really 'me' to move in with a man I hardly knew?

'Open up your options, Karen, your life doesn't have to just be in Australia,' he said.

Two days later I was on my way to LA. Once again I understood that life's journey is made of pivotal moments. Moments which pass at lightning pace. As quickly as they flash by, there are times when you know the instant they happen that your life has changed. I knew that when Mum left. These pivotal moments are especially clear when you suffer loss, but not so obvious at other times.

My love affair with New York began because of Ron. I think that our time together was crucial for me. I knew that my experience in the Big Apple could never be replicated, but he had planted a seed in my mind about New York which would change my life. I didn't quite know how it would change my life, I just knew that it would.

Our intense conversation at dinner and stroll up Fifth Avenue was followed by a kiss goodbye and a parting of the ways. The moment was lost as quickly as it had come and I was in a yellow cab on my way back to JFK, all the way trying to dismiss my anxieties about returning home to Australia.

My exchange year would soon be over and my new friends and the cities I'd grown to love would be fleeting moments that would fill the treasure box in my mind and become happy memories.

Chapter 11
Handbags and Gladrags

'Open your options, Karen, your life doesn't have to just be in Australia.'

Ron's words kept ringing in my ears. I flew to LA, the first stop on my homeward journey to Australia, contemplating my future. I was thinking about Ron and considering his invitations. I couldn't see how I could get back to the East Coast for the Presidential Inauguration nor could I imagine myself moving into his pied-à-tierre—but I could see myself living in America. He had planted a seed.

On a lark, while visiting Lisa in LA, I stopped into an employment agency in Beverly Hills. The glossy matron on duty told me that a former supermodel who was the wife of a rock and roll legend, was looking for a nanny.

'I'm a teacher,' I said.

She smiled. 'That's a plus.'

I piloted Lisa's elderly BMW along Mulholland Drive to a gated community in zip code 90210, where the celebrity couple lived with their two young children in a mansion set on acres of rolling lawn. His wife, dressed in jeans and a T-shirt, as casual in manner as she was in dress, sat with me in her sunny parlour as her two-year-old son and four-year-old daughter played nearby using an old cardboard box as a cubby house. Dad tinkered away in the background.

We chatted politely and laughed that I couldn't find the front door of her mansion and had stood on the side porch knocking on the glass roller doors trying to get in for the interview. When talk turned to nannying, she was enthusiastic about my ideas for academic and art projects. A few days before my Qantas flight home and return to life in the 'burbs', I was offered the job—but first I had to get a work visa. My new boss said she'd take care of that.

I returned to Oz and resumed teaching at St Luke's until the visa arrived. I had fulfilled the terms of my exchange contract by going back to my old job, even if it was for just a few months. But I hadn't taken the time I needed to face my anxieties about going home and understanding myself. Instead, I buzzed around, changed my external surroundings and in doing so placed a band-aid on my feelings, masking them with all the pretense that went with my next exciting adventure.

The school year began as normal. I was teaching Grade Four and was keen to meet my new students on the first day and tell them about my overseas adventures. The first face I saw peeping around the corner that warm February morning was Amy's. She greeted me with a bright smile and a bear hug. It was a blessing to see her. I had been told the day before when I checked my class list to expect a visit from Amy—who I loved so much—and her mother, Colleen.

When my visa came through a couple of months later the school asked me to resign. No longer would they retain a position for me should the nanny experiment fail and I elect to return to Australia. The 'open door' they had kept for me in the past was closed. There was a new principal at St Luke's. I had not worked for him before, nor had I proven myself to him. He was not thrilled about my new job and annoyed that I wanted to leave in March—so early in the new school year. I felt very torn but also understood the resilience of children and I knew that they would survive.

Of all the children I had taught in my seven years at St Luke's the hardest one to leave was Amy. The irony was that it was from her mother that I got most of my support. Colleen told me to follow my dreams because life was too short and that Amy would be fine. I cried when I said goodbye to my little friend and so did she. I wondered if I'd ever teach a child like her again. I loved her with all my heart—as if she were my own.

A few days later I flew back to LA, my suitcases filled with clothing and clandestine meds.

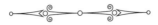

The rock-and-roll legend's manager and his wife collected me at LAX and I moved into their mansion in Beverly Hills. Perched on bedrock at the top of the Hollywood Hills, the home was palatial, elegant and cool. As we entered the grounds and drove up the long driveway, even though it was my second visit, I gazed around wide eyed and tried to take it all in. The driveway ended with a loop around a focal point—a circular, landscaped island garden bed surrounded by sandstone pavers.

The house was large with at least seven or eight bedrooms, but it still had a homely feel. Family photos adorned the cabinets, thoughtfully chosen artwork decorated the walls along the spiral staircases and kids' toys were strewn around the porches and the swimming pool. Later, the family would allow me to take regular therapeutic swims in their pool. A plastic five-foot high children's playhouse rested on the manicured lawns among the rose bushes.

As the manager parked the car I wondered what I was doing in this rock-and-roll household. I was a *teacher*, as I'd proudly declared at the employment agency. Why would I want to be a nursemaid and nanny?

A friend suggested that I was getting a chance to see what it was like to be a mum—and I bristled. She'd hit too close to home. Lately I'd been on the sidelines of many weddings and christenings. I was a godmother four times and my brother, Steve, and his wife, Trudy, were so proud of their sons. I wanted my nephews to have my children to play with in the backyard one day. At age 32, with my space-shuttle hip, signs of crippling RA in my hands and a string of unhappy romances behind me, I began to doubt my body's ability to carry a child.

Was I role-playing in my new gated life?

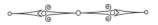

The new job started well. My glamorous supermodel boss drove us to a school supplies store and bought armloads of classroom goodies

I selected—posters of the alphabet, numbers and phonics; an easel and paints; buckets of chalk; board games; writing supplies and books. I redecorated her children's playroom and it was there that she greeted me on the first night with a chilled glass of white wine. She liked my idea of displaying the kids' art, even if the pictures were stick figures with missing feet, hands and fingers. Despite the missing body parts, their oldest child never forgot to draw each member of her family. Sometimes this was just her mum, dad and brother and other times it included her stepbrothers and stepsisters.

The rock-and-roll legend had encouraged this sibling love and the 'nest' seemed to be built around a true spirit of understanding and affection for each other. The children from his former marriage had their own bedrooms and were always welcome in the home he shared with his new family.

During the weekdays I lived upstairs with the family in the main part of the mansion which had dramatic views of the Hollywood Hills. I had been assigned a bedroom adjoining the son's, which meant that I could get up and care for him when he called 'Kaz' in the middle of the night. The sound of him crying out for me in the still of the night made me feel like a mum. I didn't mind getting up for him. One thing I had learnt from teaching was that it is not hard to love other people's children. I was a novice at the motherly role, however, and remember the first time I changed his diaper I put it on back to front. It took a while for him to warm to me, but when I heard him calling my name at night I knew that he was secure and that the connection would grow.

His sister had a harder time with me as the new nanny. The transition from the last nanny to the new was difficult for her because she was older—but I understood that. Some of the staff, like the housekeepers, had happily worked for the rock and roll legend for many years and so they had won his daughter's trust. I had to earn it. I could see that this was her way of controlling her surroundings. Our relationship would take a little time but I couldn't blame her. Like all children she craved the familiar.

I was determined to be the magical nanny who would make a difference in the children's lives. A regular Mary Poppins was my plan. I decided to get the children to work on a project with me. I thought if we knuckled down as a team it would form a greater bond. On Mother's Day, a month after I arrived, we surprised supermodel mum with a performance of *Three Billy Goats Gruff*. The children and I painted a backdrop and set up a makeshift stage on the tennis court. Always a good sport, the rock and roll legend made a hilariously rowdy troll as he shouted gruffly: 'Who's that walking over my bridge?' while sitting under a table on the concrete court. The kids and I were dressed up as billy goats while mum applauded vigorously—along with the housekeepers who made up the rest of the audience.

The project worked and helped me connect with the children. I loved it because I was using my teaching skills and they entered into the spirit of it all because it was fun. This celebrity couple were 'hands-on' parents and were around daily. Supermodel mum would often drive her daughter to school and her sister, who also lived at the mansion, helped shuttle the kids to care and after-school activities. The two stunning blonde sisters reminded me of surfer chicks from Oz. They were suntanned, 'outdoorsy' types who loved to go to spinning classes together and hike the Hollywood Hills. Surprisingly, the supermodel's sister was a bit of a Sun Goddess. One night when we were out together in Santa Monica I heard a bar tender say: 'I've got two words for you: sun block.'

She was a good sport and laughed it off.

The celebrity mum spent her days working on projects, taking French classes with a private tutor, getting the odd massage, hanging out with the kids and her sister and doing the odd bit of 'grooming maintenance'. It seemed like she preferred the hairdresser, seamstress and masseuse to do home visits. Why not I thought—I would too if I could.

Rocker dad spent his days with his children—there were five at the time—as well as with his trains and toy soldiers. He played soccer in the garden with his son at every opportunity. His hobby is model trains and he dedicated half of the top floor of his house to them. A large model train set meandered its way through bubbling brooks, hills, forests and mountains frosted with snow and was complete

147

with a cloud-painted backdrop. This provided him with his escape. Another was the regular Saturday morning soccer and weekday team practice.

One day the rock and roll legend and I shared an afternoon by the pool where he talked about soccer and I realised how close the game was to his heart. He described it as physical, skillful, exciting and a truly global sport.

'I could have played soccer at the elite level. I had to make the choice between my music and professional soccer. I think I made the right choice,' he said.

I knew without doubt that he had done that. His music had given so many people so much joy. I had liked his music before I was appointed a family staff member, but, as I got to know him I was more inclined to listen to it. I wanted to understand him better. He proved to be an uncomplicated person with a great sense of humour and a big heart. He liked to joke about himself, was nostalgic at times and he wanted the best for his children. He often talked to me about schooling for his eldest son and believed in trying to teach his kids about the value of money. This was reinforced by his belief that they should earn their weekly allowance. Overall I got the impression that the perfect day for this legend was simple: it was time by the pool, an afternoon game of soccer and dinner with family and friends in the evening. The way he treated his wife, family and employees was more important to him than what he did for a living, and sharing a meal with his wife and family and creating loving memories together was, to him, what life was all about.

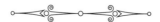

My RA continued to flicker in the background like a dim reminder that it could abruptly take control of my life. There was always pain and a hint that it was lurking and waiting to pounce like a tiger on its prey, but I was in denial and refused to listen to the warning signs my body was giving me. I told myself I was feeling normal and so I *was* normal. But, again, I was deluding myself.

As I began to flare more frequently, I began to feel the burden of hiding my disease. Negative thoughts bubbled to the surface and I was having trouble controlling them. I told myself I was lonely and that I was just living vicariously through this Hollywood couple. Even though I felt a connection and an obligation to the family, the increasing pain from my RA and the energy it took to fight the pain disempowered me. I struggled with this negativity and the energy required to stop these thoughts.

There were other triggers as well. My looming 33rd birthday and Lisa's motherhood didn't help. I began to question my decision to take the job. And if a relationship with Ron Silver had been part of my original motivation to move to LA, it hadn't worked, as I'd only seen him once since I had become a 'rock'n roll nanny'.

I began to write therapeutic letters home to Mum; it was the only way I could truly 'voice' how I felt. As I wrote I reflected on the decisions I'd made and the lifestyle of celebrities of this magnitude.

22 May 1997

Dear Mum,

It's 9 p.m. and finally the lights are out. It took a while to get the kids down tonight. I know this is a good learning experience for me and good preparation for motherhood. Every day I understand you better, Mum. We are in West Palm Beach, Florida and I have Monaco, the QE2 and the French Riviera to look forward to over the summer. But I feel like crying and I really need to talk to you. There are many times lately that I am left pondering whether I made the right choice to leave Amy and my class. I think of Amy often and wonder if she has adjusted to my absence. I also worry about her health because I've heard she's been in and out of hospital a lot since I left. I wonder about my decision to give up teaching, a career I love, to do this nannying job. I am also finding the hours long and it is physically very demanding. I guess that's what it is really like to be a mum—exhausting!

Yes, the lifestyle is opulent and the travel is nice. I've now seen the true power of money and it is amazing. But the price this family pays for it is high. As an observer of this lifestyle, I think if ever I had the choice, 'to have or to have not', I would not choose fame and fortune over an existence like say, yours, Mum, or Steve and Trudy's. You can still do basically all that you

want to and you're not living in a fish bowl. I feel bad for them at times and
for the kids.

Finding the opportunity to send this will be hard, but I guess I feel better for
just having written my feelings down now. I'm looking forward to sharing
some good times with you again soon.

Love you lots,

Kaz

A letter from Mum, following a tearful telephone call, was so
warming and reassuring.

24 May 1997

My Darling Kaz and Special Friend,

I am so glad I was able to get back to you shortly after you called and
hope I was of some help to you. My immediate reaction was to want to
put my arms around you and hold you tight. Being a mum, or in your case
a 'pseudo' mum takes a terrific amount of energy and most of all good
health. I get so angry when I think that the latter has passed you by, but
we can't change that, only work to make it easier. Try and be really positive
about the good points of your new job and don't focus on the negative. The
negatives are obviously loneliness, boredom, lack of people your own age,
mental stimulation and a lack of private time. But I think if you were to
compare that to where you used to live in Sydney and the same old places you
used to go to, this situation would have to come out on top. As far as your
seven years towards long service leave is concerned, don't worry about that
at all. If you had the three months off with paid leave you'd be travelling
anyway and that's what you're doing now. The places you live in and how
you travel must surely be above the average and, Kaz, the money is good.
However, nothing absolutely nothing is worth your happiness. Don't give in
because of boredom, because the commitment to this family really deserves to
be honoured even though it may not be quite what you expected. But should
anything detrimental affect your health then you should think about your
options.

Being a mum requires sacrifices too. Often loneliness during the day, or
boredom at home, affects full-time mums badly. Yes they have a partner to
come home to them at the end of the day, but nothing is really easy, Kaz.

Right now I think one of your biggest concerns is another birthday. At 33 you feel you need to be loved and deserve to have someone to love. You are such a giving and loving human being and that your need longs to be filled. Do you have any idea how many lonely, single people are out there in the big cities? There are thousands of people your age who long to have a genuine partner. I know there is someone for everyone and when you find your special person he will be very worthwhile.

Darling, I am going to Mass and I will pray especially for you tonight, Kaz. I love you so much all the time and I can't wait until we can spend more time together.

Love you, love you.

Take care, God bless,

Mum

PS: I am about to send this but have been thinking half the night and most of the day about your seven years at St Luke's and leaving Amy. Amy and her mum understood. Everyone in your school environment thought it was an opportunity that rarely comes along. They knew that you would have always wondered what it would have been like if you hadn't taken the chance.

The changes this job has brought to your life as someone who already had an established career are enormous, even incomprehensible. Suddenly you have two small children to care for, no friends around and no partner to go home to. I am certain in the coming months when you are familiar with the demands placed upon you and the children settle down under your care things will be a lot better. Please don't regret your decision, you can't change it anyway and you did need a change. I am sure they are very fond of you and in time, if not already, will love you. Hang in there, Kaz, you know I am always here.

God bless, take good care,

Mum.

On my birthday in June I was feted with a gourmet dinner which had been prepared especially for me by a celebrity chef. The special dining room was set with lavish cutlery, napkins and crockery. The legend and his wife gave me a gorgeous gold T-bar necklace with scattered grey and pink freshwater pearls and tiny glass beads. This present was accompanied by another one; an oriental cloth journal.

But the best gift of all was when the whole family joined me for dinner and my rock and roll boss sang a funky version of 'Happy Birthday'.

The moment was memorable and sweet—bittersweet. I was surrounded by opulence, living the glam travel life I'd dreamed of as a teen and earning more money than I ever had as a teacher.

A few days earlier I had received the news that Amy had died and none of it mattered any more. I was devastated. She died on my mother's birthday and was buried on mine. She left us and went to a place where she could be pain-free. Death had given Amy's soul the freedom it deserved to move on to another level. But for those left behind it was hard to see her go. The world seemed a lonelier place without 'Our Amy'.

Amy's peace with her own fate gave me more strength to be at peace with mine. She seemed to understand her destiny and had the calmness of a person who was not scared about being sick, but accepted that her illness was a condition of her living.

Not long after the news of Amy's death I received a letter from her mother.

Dear Karen,

I hope this letter finds you well and caring for yourself. I know how hard it must be for you at this time, being apart from your family and your many friends.

I wanted to let you know that although Amy's passing was sudden, it was peaceful and pain-free. As with everything in Amy's life, she did it her way and in her own time, making quite sure that everyone had time to say their goodbyes.

I know in my heart that Amy was ready to make the journey 'home' and that she is now at peace. Amy's life was short but it was certainly filled with joy and loving. For one so small and vulnerable she left her mark on this world. Many people have written many wonderful words about Amy, including yourself. A friend wrote this and I would like to share it with you! 'Don't grieve because I've gone, just be happy I was there.' It warms my heart to know that Amy was loved by so many people. You will always remain in my heart with a great affection, not only for all you gave to Amy as her teacher,

*but also for the love you gave her as her friend and for all the support you
gave to me. Amy's final resting place is beautiful. She lies in the shade of a
very old elm tree close to a playing field where she can hear the children play.
Amy's passing has created a great void in many lives, none so great as my
own, but I am sure that she is now the 'boss' in Heaven.*

*Thank you, Karen, for all that you gave to both Amy and myself. Please
always be kind to yourself and take care. May God bless you always and
know that Amy will always watch over you.*

Yours in peace and with love

Colleen—'Amy's Mum'.

I was heartbroken about Amy's death and I wondered why the
world was so unfair. I didn't ever tell my employers—I don't know
why. I think I needed to mourn her and feel the loss alone. They did
seem to sense that I was unhappy. Because of my sadness I found
it difficult to summon up the energy I needed for the children. I
thought a lot about the good fortune of the children in my care.
They had good health, good looks and exceedingly wealthy parents.
To be born into such a position was powerful—and lucky, I guess.
Why then was there such pain for a little soul like Amy? Or was
this the wrong way to view things? She wasn't blessed with good
health, but Amy was blessed with the gift of being able to deeply
touch the heart of every child or adult she ever met. Her impact was
everlasting.

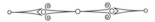

That summer we spent time at the family's ocean-front house in
West Palm Beach. We flew to New York, sailed to England on the
QE2, then choppered from the dockside to their estate in Essex.
It didn't really matter where we were because with this superstar
level of fame it was often only the 'four walls' the family got to see
anyway.

The estates had been set up so that there was little need to leave
for anything. Dining out was a popular past time, but even that had
a price. The family and I were eating at the Ritz Carlton in West

153

Palm Beach when we were waylaid by a group of 50-plus women on a girls' night out. With a few champagnes under their belts they had Dutch courage and approached the table. This was fine and the rocker was a gentleman, but the number of the group started to expand and we had to grab the kids and disappear fast. Model mum, relieved to be in the car, told the driver:

'Quick, just drive.'

Another time when he was minding his own business and walking through an airport terminal a bystander began shouting obscenities at him: 'You can't sing. You're just a drug pusher,' he barked.

The jealousy and envy of members of the public astounded me. I couldn't fathom that people could be so rude and disrespectful. As regular people out of the spotlight, I don't think we understand that at all. It is fair to say that, as a high-profile celebrity, he goes to places where he feels protected; I guess he has to. That was one of the reasons why he loved his yearly cruise on the *QE2*. He could take his extended families, dine in the VIP section and be left alone.

After the *QE2* cruise and chopper trip from the port we settled into a Georgian manor house with its own staff, plus a pair of chefs flown in from LA.

The manor sat in the shade of English oaks and muscular-stemmed hornbeams of Epping Forest where the royals used to chase stags at Christmas in days gone by. Opened by Queen Victoria in 1882 as a Royal Forest it had become a wooded sanctuary for the moneyed people of the world. The rocker's property sat on some hundred acres of pristine woodland with separate guest quarters, a pool, a lagoon, a stable for the horses and another separate house for the stable manager.

This legend was most proud of the professional quality of his football pitch where he sometimes held mini tournaments to feed his other passion. Trophies adorned the bar where he would sometimes ask players back for a drink after a run around the pitch. I could tell that he got great pleasure from showing me around the property.

Before I was able to fully relax and take the days off that I knew I deserved, having worked 24/7 for ten days, I was called into the office by my supermodel boss.

'When we were in the helicopter you did not seem to have a "sense of the occasion", Karen. I'd like to know why.'

I didn't know what to say. I knew she was right. Flying over London in a helicopter had been unbelievably beautiful, but I was physically and emotionally exhausted. I was tired from working, I was flaring and I was still grieving for Amy. On the *QE2*, after the kids had gone to bed, I'd spent nights in the cabin quietly writing to Colleen and my mum as a way of overcoming my grief.

I tried to explain away my pain by saying I was tired. Perhaps I should have told her then about Amy and perhaps I should have told her about my RA too. But I didn't. It was wrong of me not to explain because in doing that I compromised my responsibilities as the children's nanny. I should have told her in that moment, for the sake of her kids because I am quite sure she would have understood.

The summer days were spent at Epping, in Essex county, mainly with the youngest son, hanging out playing soccer on the private pitch, rowing around the lagoon and trying to keep him occupied. I began to feel that we were bonding. The things he loved to do: play soccer and play with trains, were really a window into his dad's world. The daughter's love of the Spice Girls, her pretend performances and her ballet also offered a window into her parents' world—her mum had loved ballet as a child too.

We had been in Epping a few weeks and I started to have sharp pains in my lower back. I had not been feeling very well for several days, but I was trying to 'lift my game' and the last thing I wanted to do was admit that I was sick and ask for time off to go to the doctor. I tried to ignore the way I was feeling and push through it, after all I'd done that so many times before. But things came to a head after a night of high temperatures, passing blood in my urine and a morning of working with severe pain. I simply could not ignore the throbbing pain in my back any longer. I sheepishly asked if I could use the car to go to see a doctor. They didn't hesitate.

Unfortunately, the doctor took one look at me and said: 'You have a severe kidney infection and you're suffering from exhaustion. You need to be admitted to hospital now. You can't drive the car home, an ambulance will take you. I will call the manor and let them know.'

I was forced to leave their car at the surgery. They were told to come and pick up it up and I was admitted into the local public hospital using my Medicare card. The family called for updates and came to visit me, but somehow I knew, as I lay looking into their daughter's big brown eyes, that it would be better for the children if I resigned. I knew that my compromised immune system caused by the RA medication had fuelled my kidney infection and I was scared that something bad would happen again.

My health was again 'predictably unpredictable' and I couldn't draw the rock and roll legend, his wife and their kids into that. They needed a nanny who they could rely on to be there one hundred per cent of the time. I knew that I was making the responsible decision but I was very distressed that once again the disease had won. I felt like I'd failed at my first opportunity to be a mum and I questioned if I'd ever be able to manage a family of my own.

I lay in the public ward of the English hospital knowing the job was over, but not yet grasping how I was going to tell my boss. I felt like I had just bonded with the kids and I'd dreamed of being different from the other nannies and about making a real difference to their lives. I had failed. Somehow I found the courage and resigned from my hospital bed. I wanted to give them as much time as possible to find a replacement.

They understood and said that they wouldn't cancel my US visa immediately so that I could figure out when it would be best for me to travel home. They swung into action to find a new nanny and I tried to focus on getting well again.

Mum called me at the hospital morning and night. I'd count down the hours in between our conversations. I was terribly depressed but she was there for me again. Our relationship was now healed. It felt good.

I wrote her a letter from my hospital bed.

6 July, 1997

Dear Mum,

Hi! It's just half an hour until your call. What would I do without you? I just wanted to let you know how much your support has meant to me. Thank you. I love you so much and will always be there for you too.

This hospital (more like an institution) is really quite unbelievable, it is full of characters. Imagine this. Tonight I was with two 74-year-olds in the common room watching Coronation Street. *The conversation between them began like this:*

'How old are you?'

'I'm not quite sure, I really can't remember.'

'I was born in 1923.'

'So was I.'

Finally, I settled myself back into my bed, which is in a room with seven others. I commented on the terrible food to one of them. The obese lady opposite replied in her thick, northern English accent: 'I was about six and a half stone until I was 30, then one night I went to bed and when I woke up I was a few stone heavier. I've been like that ever since.'

Then there's the other 25-stone, toothless lady with a foghorn voice and the woman who doesn't like me because the Aussies win the cricket all the time. This is my life right now and these are the people with whom I share my bedroom. How quickly things can change!

Five minutes till you call, Mum. Can't wait, your calls keep me going. Otherwise I would feel so alone. There's been no word from the estate today, but I understand that.

With love from much too far away,

Kaz

Once I was out of hospital and back with the family on their estate, I needed to diarise the events of the past couple of months.

13 July: It's the night before we leave London for LA, I have a ten-hour flight and 12 straight days of work ahead of me and then that's it. My life will change again. I don't know why God led me on this path except that I've learned a lot about life.

Maturity makes this rock and roll legend a very nice man. He loves his wife dearly and you can see he just wants to please her and make her happy. He sent her flowers recently that were six feet tall. The card congratulated his model wife for a 'great audition'. He is a good man.

During the past four months I've had periods of extreme loneliness, boredom, despair, frustration, stress and anxiety. It'll hit me back in LA when I move out of the rocker's home and am back at Lisa's in Van Nuys. My life seems like it is such a mess now. But I'm praying for guidance from above and from Amy. Maybe I'll be led to a family and a husband of my own. It surely must be my turn. I'll always be grateful to the family for this experience and the lessons I've learned about fame. Strangely, they reminded me about the value of family.

So will it be LA for six months or home to Australia in a few weeks and back to my family and friends and the career I love? We'll see...

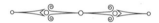

I left the hills of Hollywood within a month. The rocker loaded me up with signed CDs and photographs, and his wife and the kids posed for farewell photos. Saying goodbye to the children was hard, but I found comfort in the knowledge that I'd made the right decision for them. Before I knew it I was back home in Sydney and happy to be there.

While in LA, I'd been offered a job by my old boss, John. I took the relief teaching position at his new school which was in a low socio–economic area. The gulf between the world I had just left and the one I had barrelled into was amazing. Suddenly I was faced with the reality of a world which can be cruel. I saw how hard it was for poorer children to work their way out of their destiny.

As I turned my back on the celebrity lifestyle, I was grateful to this rock and roll legend that he had taught me about the gift of time. He'd taught me that spending time with family and friends was something that could not be bought and that family was more valuable than 'handbags and gladrags'. Once I understood that, I knew home was exactly where I needed to be.

Chapter 12
Angel On My Shoulder

When I resigned from my position with the rocker and his wife and returned to Australia, I knew that I'd made my last detour from the classroom.

It became abundantly clear to me that I had plenty to offer my pupils—perception and awareness, hope and encouragement, even love. The lessons my body had forced on me—perseverance and self-acceptance—honed my sensitivity to the individual struggles of my students for academic achievement and peer approval.

Some young children have a huge capacity to learn quickly; others, even with expert help, can't help stumbling along the way. The physical challenges I'd faced for almost two decades had taught me how to put distractions aside and focus on what can be accomplished each day. I knew I could keep pace and provide daily challenges for the best brains in my classroom, while being an effective, gentle safety net for the less talented kids.

I completed the year as a relief teacher and then took a job teaching first grade at a Sacred Heart Catholic school. It was in a superb location—the waterside suburb of Rose Bay—and the curriculum included the religious lessons I'd been given as a child. I planted my roots right there, almost 1000 km from where I'd grown up. I spent time with my brother and his family who were also living in Sydney and often flew interstate to visit my parents. I loved living a street from the ocean in Sydney's eastern suburbs and always stopped at Tamarama Beach on the drive home from work to take in the view and chill out from the school day. A ritual swim in the sea pool at Coogee capped each glorious day.

Tamarama beach, or 'Glamourama' as the locals called it because of the gorgeous Aussie girls who sunbathe there, was nature's gift. It's a small picture-perfect ocean beach nestled in amongst the headlands, parks and stunning homes. I never risked swimming there because of the rips—it's the most dangerous patrolled beach in New South Wales—but I loved to gaze out to sea, with the wind blowing in my face and drink in all the beauty around me. This was the one time in the day that I could sit and think of nothing—like Wordsworth celebrated in his poem *Daffodils*: 'In vacant or in pensive mood'. After a few minutes of allowing my mind to go totally blank I would feel a sense of invigoration. It was as if being with nature reinvigorated me. I seemed to have an 'energy account' and, when I took the time to make 'nature deposits' I became a better person and a better teacher.

Happiness in my work and serenity in my surroundings helped me in my efforts to control my disease, but RA is a cunning customer, always looking to dent the protective shield provided by stress management and medication. The fear of a flare or sudden return to hospital was never far away.

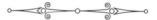

The inevitable happened in September 1998. Instead of heading south to Melbourne for the Australian Rules Grand Final I found myself in trouble again. Mum flew to my bedside, as usual. After having more bilateral knee aspirations and cortisone injections following an RA flare I was rushed to hospital with suspected septic arthritis. Caused by bacteria, septic arthritis can lead to serious infection of the joints and multiple organ dysfunction.

My body had failed me again. Intravenous antibiotics were pumped into me, my knees were re-aspirated and an arthroscopic operation performed. With the intravenous bottle suspended over me I focused on the constant dripping of the antibiotics into the tube that led to my vein and wondered how I'd ended up in hospital again. Could it have been the cut on my leg that I suffered while on the playground supervising the children? I didn't have time to clean it properly before going back to my classroom. How could I know? Was my immune system really that depleted? The rhythmic droplets of antibiotics reminded me of a ticking metronome, slicing up time. For me, time couldn't go quickly enough. I couldn't wait to get out of there. After ten days and no growth of organisms in my culture I was released from hospital back into the world of the healthy.

The disturbing aspect of being in hospital was that RA wasn't my only health issue. This was the third time I had been admitted because of an infection I had contracted. It pointed to the fact that my immune system was compromised. My body simply could not deal with infections. All this had been triggered by my RA drugs which wiped out one problem but introduced another by stripping my body of its ability to protect itself.

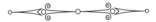

It was December 1999. Libby and I decided to take a millennium cruise out of Miami and around the Bahamas during our school holidays. It was a few days into the year 2000 and Libby and I were playing the tourists in New York. We positioned ourselves in Times Square on West 47th Street thinking we were in the heart of it all. We thought our 1920s vintage hotel was in a 'prime location' with a Starbucks on the corner and the Barrymore Theatre across the road.

New York continued to romance me. On our last night in the city we splurged and went for a drink at The View restaurant overlooking Times Square. Panoramic views of New York—360 degrees—surrounded us. Yet again I was enchanted by the charm of the city and overwhelmed by the magic of the Chrysler Building. The sights invigorated me and brought back to vivid life every dreamy image and memory I had of New York City. It was then that I decided that this was where I wanted to live.

After this taste of Gotham I'd now seen enough of the world to know that my own personal Emerald City wasn't to be found in Oz. I'd fallen for New York for all the usual reasons—its energy, its multiplicity, its sense of boundless opportunity. Despite my nagging health issues, I focused on getting a job in the Big Apple.

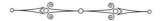

A few semesters later, on a lovely summer's day in 2000, I stood on the roof deck of the United Nations International School with the administrator in charge of recruiting. Months of daily phone calls to his office (made at midnight my time from Sydney) had paid off. When I'd learnt from his secretary that he received more than 3000 applications from teachers every year, I booked a flight to New York the day before my scheduled phone interview and showed up in person instead.

We watched the tall ships parade down the East River. I kept my bent fingers out of sight. And, though I felt I had presented my person and my qualifications in the best possible way, I returned to Sydney not knowing if the trip had been worthwhile. To my delight I was offered a job within a few weeks.

My achievement was sidelined by the saddest of happenings. The same day that I received the good news, the family was told that Trudy, Steve's wonderful wife and the mother of his two beautiful sons, had bowel cancer.

The grim reality of this moment seized us all. In the blink of an eye Trudy's world had changed and our world had also changed. The outlook seemed exhausting. First there was the operation to remove the diseased portion of Trudy's bowel and then she would have to start a six-month treatment of chemotherapy as a precautionary measure. The boys were four and six and they needed their mum. How could this be happening? We were all devastated but, as a family, we rallied and got busy. We rolled up our sleeves, gathered together close relatives to help and planned our course of action.

For me it was very painful to see the fear on Trudy's face as she went through the chemotherapy sessions. I think I understood this type of fear because of my disease. It was a fear that screamed out loud and clear: 'Something is happening to me and it's out of my control'.

After the first round of chemotherapy I believe Trudy's continuing fear was born out of dread, rather than the unknown. She knew what to expect with each session and there was no escape, like a nightmare that wouldn't end. The thought of it must have haunted her and lingered in the background, hovering like storm clouds overhead. The chemo was battering her and she couldn't run away. Her worst fear was the thought of not being around to see her boys grow up—but she marshalled all her life force and from it drew reserves of strength even she didn't know existed within her. She did that with Steve's help. Together they would have no negative talk about the future.

Secretly my mind played through many scenarios for them and their boys and I was angst-ridden over my immediate future—to take the job in New York, or stay in Sydney where I could be of help. What was I to do? How could I possibly turn my back on my brother when he needed me so badly? How could I accept the UN job now?

I turned to Steve for advice. As always, he was positive. He would handle it. Steve never doubted that Trudy would be well again and was certain that he could cope with flying planes, looking after a sick wife and caring for two young, energetic boys. I wasn't convinced. He had been my rock and I wanted to be his. We had many conversations and each time Steve became more and more adamant that my life should not stop because of Trudy's cancer and that I should accept the job. I did. But I struggled over what to do more than they ever knew.

Trudy's treatment had become part of the family's daily rhythm. Hospital visits, doctors visits, test results and Trudy's absence at school dismissal time had almost become commonplace. I decided that I would do all that I could to help before I left for New York. Sometimes I would collect the kids from school and stay on to help with house cleaning and cooking before returning home late at night to continue packing for New York. We all pitched in and Steve took time off work to care for his ailing wife.

After the first couple of chemo infusions Trudy was constantly sick—so sick that she could no longer get up the stairs to the bedroom she shared with Steve. A makeshift bedroom was set up in the living room. When I visited her I saw a woman who was a mere shadow of the sister-in-law I'd known. Unable to face food, she was painfully thin and fragile. It seemed like her body was surrendering.

The attack of pneumonia which I had suffered some years before had taught me what it meant to struggle with the fragility of life and to face one's own mortality. As I sat by Trudy's pull-out bed staring across the antique wooden table around which we'd all shared Christmas dinner less than a year before, her hand reached for mine. Gripping me tightly she locked her pale blue eyes with mine and announced: 'I *will* be around for my boys. I might get sicker before I get better, but I *will* be around for my boys.'

It was a declaration of war. There was no hesitation, no denial and no bargaining—just an acceptance that the brawl between her and the cancer was on.

My brother's insistence that my life shouldn't stop empowered me with the courage I needed to walk away from him when I felt his world was in crisis. A week or so before I left Australia Steve gave me a card. On the front of it was a map of the world. The oceans were gold and the countries left white. Australia was positioned towards the front. The card's words were written in a comical font: *No matter where you are…We still seem close.*

Inside the card Steve had written:

> *Kaz,*
> *You are the only person in the world who I can call my sister. Since we were little children we've always been together supporting one another. I've been truly blessed to have someone as special as you in my life. I greatly respect your courage, talent, persistence and compassion. Your beauty shines through your heart to all those you touch. Thank you for shining on me. As hard as I try, my words cannot express how much you mean to me. I am so very proud of you. I miss you already. Remember you are just a day's flight away. Thank you for loving me and my family back. My family is your family. Lots of love from your big brother,*
> *Steve.*

True to his character Steve did not mention his own pain in the card or his needs. He just encouraged me to follow my dream and convinced me that he and his family would be fine.

It was with mixed emotions that I packed up my house and stored my belongings. By the end of August I was back in New York, my suitcases unpacked for a one-year teaching position at the United Nations school. I had high hopes, hidden fears and great sadness about leaving my family, but particularly leaving Steve when his life was upside-down.

I knew I could handle the job at the International School and I was thrilled to get a chance to live in the city I loved. But, coming through customs with a suitcase full of medicine, I also worried that my body would betray me. As I shuffled to the luggage carousel in JFK airport, diplomatic visa in hand, I wondered if I could pull off my charade. Though I'd brought enough medicine to last till the end of the school year, I knew my health could change as quickly as New York weather.

If my RA took a turn for the worse, I'd have to find a doctor to give me a high-dose cortisone shot in an ailing joint. But what if I sailed through my trial year at the UN school and was offered another year's work? Or better yet, a permanent position? When would the time come—and what would it cost me—to tell my employers I had RA? I felt the burden of my secret, but I knew I was a good teacher and I wanted to be judged for that. So long as I was doing my job well I didn't feel obligated to tell my employer anything about my RA. If something went wrong then I would expose my vulnerability. My experience with the celebrity family had taught me that this was the right course of action. I just hoped my health would hold out until I had proved my value so that my employer wouldn't think I was counterfeit stock.

My hopes were high as I prepared to present myself to my new colleagues as an able-bodied, fun-loving Aussie. *G'day!*

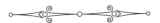

I arrived in Gotham and moved straight into my 'Ghostbuster' Gothic-style apartment building which my new boss had arranged for me. I was greeted and helped with my luggage by a uniformed doorman. Wow, I thought, how cool is this? A doorman, just like the movies, just like at Ron's.

The lobby was Tudor style. It was filled with stained-glass windows, grey slate tiles and antique furniture. I couldn't wait to get inside my new apartment. Even though I'd been told it was a 'studio' apartment, the adjective meant nothing to me. I caught the elevator to the fourth floor and strolled down the corridor, dizzy with anticipation—as well as seriously jetlagged. I felt proud as I put the key in the door and stepped inside my Manhattan apartment…into a 'shoe box'.

My studio consisted of one room, a windowless bathroom, a pull-out sofa bed and the worst excuse for a kitchen that I'd ever seen. It was about 10 footsteps wide and 20 footsteps long with a few furry rodents as my new flat mates. The cost? US$1300 a month. A good deal? I stood there in shock. I had expected a lot more for the rent, which was going to suck up half of my wages. Welcome to New York City.

My address was Tudor City Place. Perched high on a plateau in midtown Manhattan above 42nd Street the area is a peaceful, tree-lined enclave built in the 1920s as an urban escape for city workers with a desire to live near their jobs. Gargoyles protect residents in this urban oasis; but it wasn't always utopia and my apartment was definitely no oasis. The tiny 'efficiency' apartments of Tudor City were built to rise above the stench of noxious fumes from slaughterhouses and factories along the East River where the United Nations building now stands.

Local legend has it that the 'Tudor Castles' were built for mistresses of businessmen—which would explain why the apartments are only the size of a hotel room. My only window faced inwards away from the water towards the Tudor parks; the window ledge became my place of refuge when New York City became too much.

A few days later I began my new job. I felt incredibly proud when I said: 'I teach at the United Nations International School in Manhattan'.

My classroom overlooked the East River and was big and bright. The school was founded two years after the UN was inaugurated in 1947 and now has 1500 students from more than 100 countries enrolled in classes from kindergarten through to high school. While my accent draws comments elsewhere in New York, my voice blended with an English-speaking staff of more than 70 nationalities. I found the racial and cultural diversity captivating. From the hallway outside my classroom an observer would see a tall slim blonde at the whiteboard—not young, not old. Coming closer he or she might notice my bulb-knuckled hands and a keen observer might also spot the stiffness in my movements and the shuffle in my stride. But unlike my students, whose every thought tumbles straight from their mouths, such an observer would not ask what's wrong with me. I'm grateful for that buffer zone of manners and grown-up reticence. I've used it defensively, to hide what I couldn't accept in myself and I've used it when I've reached for something I wanted but felt I might not get if the truth about me were known. Like my new job.

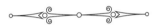

September to December was tough. Trudy continued to fight her cancer with chemicals that wrecked her body and I tore myself up thinking that Steve needed me. A new job, a foreign city and no friends—I was a fish out of water. Ron had moved on with his life and was no longer interested in me. There were nights when I sat on the window ledge and looked at the four walls and cried. Had I made a very selfish decision? Perhaps, but I was probably my harshest critic. All these things added up to stress and the strain played havoc with my RA. In a fairly short time it became evident that the aggression in my disease was winning over the drugs—I was slipping out of control. The thought that my illness would, once again, impact on my job was terrifying. Unable to afford to catch a cab to work in winter I shuffled along in the snow. My ankle joints were now constantly sore and every step I took caused unimaginable pain. Sometimes my energy was so depleted from the walk that just getting up off the chair to be closer to the kids was nearly impossible. Sometimes I propelled myself around the room on my desk chair. My hands were so inflamed that I found it difficult to write on the board and to correct the kids' work. I was always exhausted, but nobody seemed to notice. The kids were happy, they were learning and they, unknowingly, made compensations for me. Once again, I had become the master of masking my pain.

The first to know my RA secret was the young English woman who taught in the classroom across the corridor from mine. Her shoulder-length blonde hair framed an attractive face. Charlotte and I became firm friends. When she invited me to her wedding that autumn I happily accepted and was even happier when I got there and met her brother Matt.

Charlotte married Eric, her French-American beau and grandson of famed lithographer Fernand Mourlot, at a fancy Park Avenue church. Matt, who had flown in from the Cotswolds in England, gave the bride away.

Matt and Charlotte's mother and father had stayed home in Gloucestershire, both too ill to travel to America. A well-positioned cell phone on the altar lessened Charlotte's pain, while in the peacefulness of the rolling hills and valleys of the English countryside, her parents gathered around their phone to hear the priest utter the words: 'You are now husband and wife'.

From my perch on St Bartholomew's polished pew that day, I looked admiringly at my new friend's boyish brother as he proudly strode down the aisle. He had longish, dark blond hair just reaching down to touch his collar. His formal black suit hung loosely on his wiry frame and when he smiled it was with disarming shyness. Without a doubt he was 'easy on the eyes'—but ridiculously young. I estimated his age to be somewhere between 27 and 36—and he was shorter than me in the heels I'd chosen to go with my pink sequined skirt, slinky aqua top and feathered jacket.

Matt must have taken a few notes of his own. He told his big sister that he had a crush on her six-foot Aussie co-worker.

But after the joy of the wedding, Matt hit a rough patch.

His parents' health was degenerating quickly and there was no-one else to help them out in the grey Gloucestershire winter. Matt shouldered the lion's share of care-giving, though he was joined by Charlotte and his older brother shortly before they died—within weeks of one another.

The family was overwhelmed with grief. Matt later wrote to me:

'I watched as two men struggled to remove my mother's body in a green canvas body bag from my family home. That will always stay with me.'

When Charlotte returned to the UN International School she reached out and our friendship deepened. As one of the few people at work who knew about my struggles with RA and my sister-in-law's struggle with cancer, Charlotte thought I might be able to help her wrestle with the enormity of what she'd just been through. Losing both parents in a matter of weeks was a tragedy of overwhelming proportions. She knew I'd be there when she needed me and I knew she'd be there for me.

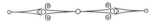

In Australia life for Steve began to improve. Trudy's chemo finished and her prognosis was good. With this news I gave myself permission to begin to enjoy New York. I started dating, a pastime that was foreign to me since Australian men don't date.

It was also time to eat vegetables. My 'kitchen' was just too small to cook in so I ate them when I dated. In my 'shoebox' I had a stovetop and a microwave but it felt as if I was cooking in my bedroom. I hated the smells that were left behind so I ate salads from Wendy's or 'dinner' with vegetables at lunchtime at the cafeteria at school.

Date, Dating, Seeing Each Other and Exclusive. The vocabulary of progressive levels of romantic interaction with the opposite sex was new to me. The one-off *Date* option was my preference. I didn't want to move up the scale to *Dating*—not yet! In New York a *Date* quite often ended with the guy putting you in a cab and in doing so the pressure was off. I loved that. No expectations. It was all over and done with at that moment unless you decided to pick up the phone and answer his calls. *Trading Up* and *Multiple Dating* were also new to me. *Trading Up* is what the midtown businessmen at the bars along Lexington Avenue are looking to do. They look to trade in their first wives for a younger, more glamorous version. *Multiple Dating* was usually done by 'wanker bankers'—men who don't get back to you for days because you're part of a cycle of women they rotate.

I quickly learned that even though Australian men were brash, you always knew where you stood with them. There was no bullshit. I started to think New York men were a waste of energy—they were not even worth 'the vegetables'.

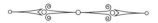

Winter blustered in to Gotham. I had heard about an Aussie expat club called *The Australian American Association* and decided I would go to their Christmas party on the first Thursday in December. I went alone. It was there that I met a group of Aussies who would become my core friends—at least until their visas expired or jobs came up in Asia or Europe. The interesting twist was that the founding members of the expat club included Sir Keith Murdoch and a man named WS Robinson, who was my paternal grandfather's boss.

WS Robinson had worked to establish himself in the Australian mining industry, frequenting far North Queensland and Western Australia in search of the elusive minerals, silver and zinc. He was the first humble director of the now-famous Conzinc Rio Tinto Corporation and the man who ignited my father's passion for flying with a gift of silver DC3 cuff links when Dad was a young boy. WS, as he was known, had a great admiration for many Americans and for the American way of life. In the late 1940s he wanted to provide a platform for transpacific economic and social alliances. In the year 2000 I was enjoying the fruits of his vision.

The first time I saw the Christmas tree lights turned on at the Rockefeller Center was with Steve and Trudy. It brought back memories of when I saw the 65-foot (20 metre) tree for the first time on my morning walk with Ron a few years before. My brother and his wife travelled the globe to celebrate Trudy's good health and even though she was still weak, we stood in the freezing cold and huddled together as Natalie Cole sang *Angel on my Shoulder* live at the Rockefeller. For the three of us the awe-inspiring illumination of the magnificent Christmas tree represented a new start for Trudy—while Steve and I privately saluted her for her victory against cancer.

A few days after they left, Dad arrived in New York for Christmas

Day—and, as always, did things that bemused me but also filled my heart with love.

'Good night then, I think I'd better go to bed, Kar.'

He tottered off towards one of only three doors in the apartment.

'No, dad, it's the closet.'

He snored happily on the sofa bed as the mouse traps clattered and I sang 'Merry Christmice' in the background. It was so good to see him, even if we were going to be cramped. After all the snow we decided to fly south for some sun. We caught a flight into Miami, hired a red convertible and drove along the narrow bridges to the Florida Keys.

In the time I'd spent in New York I'd missed dad's sense of fun and spirit; the Florida visit would be a time of bonding for us. I quietly reflected on the journey dad and I had taken together in our lives. He was a good man. I respected his honesty and perceptiveness and laughed about how gullible he was. I had never been mad at him for his absences. I'm not quite sure why…perhaps it was because I felt he handled what he could and let the rest slip. Strangely I understood his burdens and failings more than I did those of my mother. A friend once said of dad: 'Once in a while you meet people who have never been to a therapist, or read a spiritual book, but they just "get it". Your dad is one of those old souls.'

I sat quietly beside him as he drove confidently along the mile-long Keys bridges. I knew it was my chance to make the most of this precious time with my dad. The picture of Charlotte in her wedding dress with her phone pressed firmly on her ear at the altar was still etched in my mind. Our family's battles with cancer had locked our friendship in and made me appreciate them all, more than ever.

Chapter 13
Melting Pot

I was fully in the moment. It was Graduation Day for the students of the United Nations International School—Class of 2001—and we were gathered in the impressive and somewhat intimidating UN General Assembly Hall. The girl who had grown up in suburban Australia was now a player on a bigger stage. My world was no longer focused on the gorgeous beaches of Sydney's eastern suburbs and majestic Sydney Harbour with its iconic bridge and Opera House. The UN General Assembly was an awesome place to be—particularly for me because I was there as a player, a participant—not just a tourist having a look around. I felt a kinship with the world and a global perspective that I'd never encountered before as a teacher. And the kids who were graduating from the UN International School were truly blessed. Their life experience and education was second to none; their faces were confident and shining—we all felt that they were the hope of the world.

At a personal level I felt I was making giant strides. I'd seen the General Assembly a thousand times over on the television. But the privilege of sitting there, waiting for the ceremony to begin, made me feel like a kid in a candy store. My imagination took flight. In a Walter Mitty-inspired daydream I pretended I was one of the diplomats. I was representing Australia—of course—and was fluent in all six of the official languages of the UN: English, Chinese, Arabic, French, Russian and Spanish. I playfully held the cream, plastic earpiece to one ear and imagined I was listening to an interpreter repeating what I'd said—in French, or Arabic. I imagined myself working with world leaders saving children from hunger and war; framing new international laws and deploying blue-helmeted peacekeepers to help people in distress.

My flight of fancy came back to Earth as my eyes landed on the UN emblem of peace etched on a huge golden pillar dominating the backdrop to the General Assembly podium. It is a world map incorporating two olive branches—a symbol of peace and goodwill which can be traced back to ancient Greece.

It felt good to be an Australian in the General Assembly Hall that day. Fleeting thoughts of the 'Doc'—Herbert Evatt, the Australian third President of the General Assembly—crossed my mind. He had humble beginnings. He came from a working-class family in New South Wales but played an important part in the establishment of the United Nations as the Second World War drew to a close in 1945. His passion was advocating the rights of small powers. Doc Evatt's commitment to liberty was so great and his social, economic and human rights causes championed so fervently that there are parts of the UN Charter (Article 56) which are known as *The Australian Pledge*. It is a fitting tribute to one of the giants of our history.

Halfway through the Graduation Ceremony I wandered out in search of a bathroom. I tried not to attract attention as I dismissed myself from the proceedings, but it wasn't easy. My chair flipped back and I walked awkwardly out of the hall in my usual 'heel to toe' manner because of the pain in my ankles. The handicapped bathroom was closest so I decided to stop right there and use it. My thoughts came crashing down to Earth amidst a million unhappy memories when I looked at the toilet. On top of the regular seat sat a thick, plastic elevated dismountable attachment to make getting on and off the toilet easier.

Something as simple as the sight of a toilet seat tore through my psyche, snatching recollections of my hip replacement and thrusting them into the present. It was a time in my life when my RA had complete control over me. I thought of Mum lifting me off the toilet and wiping me clean; of times when my elevated toilet seat was not enough and I'd cried out to her for help and of times when I couldn't perform the most basic of physical tasks. I flicked back the pages of my past and thought about the days when I chose tops without buttons, pants without zippers and shoes without laces because of my painful hands. It seemed like a lifetime ago now.

Snapping back to reality I reminded myself I was at the UN General Assembly in New York City as an invited, even revered, guest. Had I succeeded in the face of adversity? I was enjoying life despite my illness. Had I finally accepted my disease but not become defeated by it? Almost but not quite. I knew I was getting closer. The rugged journey I'd been on to get here was just as important as this feeling of success and overcoming the odds.

I returned to the General Assembly in time to hear the keynote speaker. It was Tim Russert, a well-known political commentator in America who became famous for predicting the outcome of the 2000 Presidential election saying it would all come down to 'Florida, Florida, Florida'. Mr Russert—who, sadly, has since died—gave an inspirational speech. He talked about remembering people with AIDS, especially in Africa and the homeless throughout the world and the graduates own good fortune.

I considered the uniqueness and the ethnicities of the community he was addressing and looked around at the faces of the graduates. I saw a microcosm of the world: kids with brown hair, blonde hair, black hair and different coloured skin and facial characteristics. They spoke to each other in every language imaginable, sometimes flippantly changing from Spanish to French to English without any awareness at all that they were doing just that. The four corners of the globe seemed to come together in the General Assembly Hall and the buzz in the room was of peace and hope. Most schools I'd worked in dealt mainly with the local community. I'd never experienced such a global perspective before and I was so very proud to be a part of it.

Mr Russert's messages have continued ringing in my mind:

'Set goals and do things for others.'
'Acts of the heart make the essence of who we are.'

As they were delivered on that day I found myself nodding in agreement. Since then I've discovered the truth of them on my journey. I hoped the adults were listening as well as the students.

When I left high school none of this was in my realm of thinking. How lucky these children were.

After it was all over the graduates emerged both crying and cheering. The looks on their faces told me that they felt like they could go out and conquer the world. So, I thought, could I!

My trek had been long and hard, but the struggle was worth the feelings I had on graduation day. The nightmare of England, my hip replacement, the disease, the pain and the elevated toilet seat all shared the process. They were all part of accepting *my* disease and of calling it mine and of one day being okay with that.

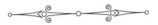

A few days later I was sitting in a dirty bus terminal on the west side of Manhattan waiting to indulge in a bit of Outlet Mall shopping. Coach, Saks Fifth Avenue, Gucci and name brands like Guess, Nine West and Gap all had shops at this mall and they threw things out for next to nothing. It was an Aussie girl's dream. The only essential I needed to buy was winter boots, so somehow I would have to control myself and curb the female temptation to buy because 'it was a good deal'. I didn't want to return home to my apartment with bags of things I didn't really need, or even like that much and shoes and tops that didn't fit but were 'nice'. Telling myself to do this, however, was always easier said than done and didn't necessarily contribute to my self-discipline.

In New York the Port Authority Terminal looks like an interstate railway station but it's for buses. Nestled in the district known as Hell's Kitchen, the Port Authority manages mass transport in the city and the bus depot is the busiest terminal in the world. West 42nd Street was unfamiliar territory. I didn't particularly like this area and found Times Square and its environs populated by seedy characters. Strangers surrounded me; the one on my left was snoring; the one on my right was belching loudly enough to make the seat vibrate and then, out of the blue, someone tapped me on my shoulder.

The man was a middle-aged African American Port Authority employee. He wore a faded blue uniform, neatly pressed and his hair was jet black and closely cropped. I was startled at first but he seemed to be a gentle soul with a kind and trustworthy face. We had a short, friendly conversation about nothing in particular, then he disappeared into one of those anonymous silver swing doors that one sees at train and bus stations. A few seconds later the door creaked open and he reappeared with a battered clipboard in one hand.

'How is your spirituality?' he asked in a soft voice.

Puzzled, I replied rather meekly: 'I wouldn't call myself spiritual, but I do have a faith.'

Then he made a statement that to me was not only profound, but magical.

'The pain you feel will ease, your hands will serve you well, the dream of your book will happen and your words will help others who are suffering. Please also spend more time with God.'

With that the gentleman double rapped the back of the yellow, plastic waiting room seat with his weathered knuckles, gathered his clipboard and strolled away, humming some old forgotten blues riff.

The message seemed like one from a friend. It took me aback and made my stomach flutter furiously because, when he spoke to me, I was actually sitting there writing notes for my book. My eyes began to billow with tears. I changed the weight uneasily from one buttock to the other and pondered the conversation as I read a Port Authority sign which hung crookedly on the wall opposite. It said: 'This is where people make the difference.'

I might have thought that I lacked spirituality in my life at that time, but I understood that this message was truly meant for me. It was time to 'make a difference'. It was time to stop, think, write and help others.

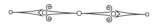

Summer began with five weeks of back-to-back visitors. My studio apartment meant I lived, slept and ate with my visitors day and night, night and day. It's not easy entertaining in a shoebox. There was barely space to walk in the apartment. One suitcase and a carry-on filled half the width of the room, when a pull-out bed, some pairs of shoes and a shopping bag or two were added, we were in a tight squeeze.

I once saw a cartoon in the *New York Times* where the guests were sleeping on the apartment building roof next to their suitcases with the Empire State Building sketched in the background. The speech bubble from the cartoon character in the apartment below said: 'If you didn't come and see me in the Middle East, don't visit me in New York.' I had to agree.

Aussies started coming out of the woodwork to visit me in New York. Pleasant phone calls from friends I hadn't seen in years were usually followed by a suitcase in hand and a knock on the door. It's kind of an Aussie mentality—get free accommodation even if it means sleeping on a wooden floor in a sleeping bag. Sometimes I'd have a guest 'turn around' time of an hour—just long enough for me to do the laundry.

My brother, of course, was one of the people I most wanted to visit. I always loved seeing him. Steve gave me a burst of positivity when I needed it most. It's his way.

He greeted me with his normal enthusiasm, a kiss hello, bear hug and a gentle question.

'Hi, Kaz, it's great to see you. Are you doing okay?'

I always held on a bit longer than him, but he'd read that need in me and hug me a bit tighter and tap me on the back saying: 'Love ya, Kaz. Miss ya, Kaz.'

Steve was good at situational comedy and loved *Seinfeld*. He quickly spotted 'Seinfeld moments' in the size of my apartment.

'Where's the bedroom? Is it through here, Kaz?'

As he was speaking he opened the kitchen pullout doors, then the bathroom door— knowing full well there was no bedroom at all.

Steve joined me and some of my new friends at a belated birthday celebration at a champagne bar. On the actual day of my 36th birthday I went to Do Hwa—an authentic Korean restaurant in Greenwich Village, a gay district with townhouses nestled amongst courtyards and winding streets.

Birthday dinners with new friends are always awkward. Everyone has different expectations. This year my hope was not to be alone.

The great thing about Aussies overseas is that they really care for one another; it's almost like there is an unspoken brotherhood culture amongst expat mates. 'Mateship' is a fundamental Australian value as deeply connected to our culture as Vegemite, the yeast-based, dark-brown, savoury spread to which most Australians are devoted—and which seems totally distasteful to the rest of the world. The concept of mateship must have developed from our convict history and was further fed by legends like that of Simpson at Gallipoli who rescued wounded soldiers time and again with his donkey. Whatever it was, the notion of looking after your mates is instilled into our value system and our national identity and is evident whenever Aussies get together—wherever they are.

The Australian parents at the UN school were no different. Our country, our sense of fun and our roguishness connected us. I didn't know Mark and Jep Lizotte, but I'd seen them in Charlotte's classroom dropping their daughter off for school. Mark was the cool dad you'd see wearing a Penguin T with roller blades slung over his shoulder. On my first Christmas in New York, Mark—whom I had known in the 1990s as pop singer Johnny Diesel—stopped by my classroom with a gift. It was his CD *Soul Lost Companion*, which he had signed:

> *To Karen*
> *Have a great holiday*
> *Cheers*
> *Mark and fam*

He had reached out to me and showed he understood what it was like to be this far from home and alone for Christmas. He was being a mate.

Then there was Venessa. I taught her daughter during my first year at the school. You can tell a lot about parents through their children. Venessa's daughter was kind, shy and beautiful as she sat in my class day after day listening carefully and doing whatever I asked of her.

On the first day of school in September, Venessa patiently waited to introduce herself and her husband Al. Al was an older dad and was very tall—making him a powerful presence in the classroom. Venessa too was hard to miss. She was stunningly glamorous with her immaculate blonde hair flowing over her designer summer floral dress. My nerves disappeared as soon as she opened her mouth.

'Good morning, Miss Ager,' she said with a strong Australian accent and a smile.

'You're an Aussie?' I asked.

'Yes, I'm a Randwick girl.'

She had been in New York for nearly 20 years and still spoke as if she was down on the beach at Coogee. I loved that. Mindful of the fine line between teacher and parent, we waited to let our friendship bloom. By Anzac Day—25 April, also Venessa's birthday—we had started to allow our Aussie connection to flower.

When I arrived at Do Hwa for my birthday celebration six weeks later, Venessa was sitting on the stool at the dark wood bar elegantly caressing the stem of her champagne flute. She had the 'it' factor and oozed sex appeal without really knowing it. Men loved her. Not long after, Charlotte arrived in her Chanel couture garb, gift in hand, looking gorgeous as always. These girls were sometimes quickly—and unfairly—judged by strangers as Fifth Avenue Princesses because they wore clothes, shoes and handbags by designers such as Prada, Gucci and Hermes. This opinion, I think, was based on nothing more than jealousy—I knew the depth of character of these women and the problems they had been through. Our connections ran deep. I felt a sense of joy as my new friends arrived to celebrate my birthday—I was so touched that they were there.

While we were chatting at the bar I glimpsed out of the corner of my eye someone arriving with a huge bouquet of flowers. It was Jep and Mark and they carried the biggest and tallest bunch of fragrant white lilies I'd ever seen. My friends were all there; my birthday night was now complete.

My belated celebration with Steve was in the Meatpackers. The Meatpackers area is all glitz, grime and cobblestone, with overpriced T-shirts, dodgy bikers' bars and only a few yellow cabs to get you home at night. The district on West 14th Street, used to be home to hundreds of slaughterhouses in the early 1900s, then became known for being controlled by the Mafia in the 1980s, only to transform itself again in the 1990s to a hipsters-hangout for the fashionable.

For some reason, turning 36 didn't faze me as much as my previous birthdays had. I didn't like getting older and being alone, but I knew I had positioned myself in a good place to meet someone and that if I wanted to have children it wasn't too late. I was confident that I was in the right place.

I did, however, feel bullied by *time* because of my RA. The disease carried with it an uncertain future and that continued to hang over me like a storm cloud threatening rain at any moment. The 'rain' I feared was damage to my joints. It was about losing them in the space of a few months because of bone degeneration. Without warning, the pain and swelling could ignite and slowly destroy my body one finger at a time. The thought of my future still made me scared, but I had come a long way and it was important to give myself credit for that.

Over the years I'd managed to work through the anger and sadness by understanding that my life was good despite my arthritis. It had taken nearly 20 years to get here, but I was beginning to accept that I had a relentless companion in my disease and that it wasn't going away. This didn't mean that I was surrendering to it. I just felt less fear about chasing my dreams and more confident about taking risks. I knew that everything was a risk because my health could swing around like the August winds in Sydney, but the chances I'd taken in Toronto, LA and now New York had worked out pretty well.

Moving to the Big Apple had empowered me and moved me forward on a track which was free of blame and defensiveness. It was true that my RA had stopped me from doing things and that it had ripped me off and taken away my twenties. I was now reclaiming the life I deserved and was opening my heart to hope.

At the champagne bar I looked around at my new friends who had joined me and marveled that my working life had overflowed into my real life. I had a *United Nations of Friends*. There to celebrate were special people from China, India, Australia, America and Sweden. In my journal I wrote: *My birthday represented to me a smaller world which is beginning to reconcile its differences.*

The year was 2001 and I, along with most of the rest of the world, was blissfully unaware of what was brewing later that year.

Trudy's steady recovery had put Steve's life back on track and gave us much to celebrate. We hit *One Flew Over the Cuckoo's Nest* on Broadway, Carnegie Hall and Wall Street. We walked around the streets of New York knowing that we would not find one answer to what it is that makes the city so special. Was it the rush of bustling people, the historical stone architecture, the roofscapes, the Madison Square Garden sporting culture, the heaving underground steam, the Central Park trees, Soho or Grand Central Station? Perhaps just an amalgam of the lot.

Steve's visit was over too quickly and before I knew it he was packing to leave. Our goodbyes were swift. They had to be. He hailed a taxi out the front of Grand Central Station, under a facade of limestone and Greek god sculptures depicting commerce, moral and mental strength. Always the trivia buff, Steve had captivated me with stories of secret underground rail tracks and clandestine elevators leading President Roosevelt to the Waldorf Astoria Hotel. But as we stood facing 42nd Street just a few blocks down from my apartment and our much-loved Chrysler Building, I felt a surge of sadness as real as a breaking wave on Bondi Beach. We had walked under the domed roof of Grand Central and through to the old Pan Am building just days before. Our time together had gone so fast. Steve had transformed my knowledge of midtown Manhattan during his visit. I even knew that a chopper had crashed on the helipad on top of the Pan Am building, killing five people in the late 1970s. He seemed to know it all and shared his knowledge with me in a gentle, brotherly way.

As I walked up the incline towards the East River and home I felt a lump in my throat so big that I could not swallow. I was overcome with love for my brother. Our farewell had triggered thoughts of our Coventry goodbye and a feeling of deep loneliness washed over me in a flood that was only mitigated by the gratitude I felt for having a brother like Steve. I had to block out at least some of these emotions for now. It was the only way I could cope with being so far from him and so far from all those I loved in Australia and all that I loved about my country.

There is an emptiness when you're used to seeing someone sit in the same seat every night, or turn the volume up on their number one song and then they're gone. It's like expecting your dog to be at the gate to greet you and he's just not there. You just expect him to jump up and when he's not around to do that—it's almost like a death. The apartment was sadly quiet and I felt so lonely without Steve. I sat on my window ledge crooking my neck so that I could look out to the red flashing lights of the Queensborough Bridge. I missed him desperately.

Steve had never described me by my arthritis like others did and like I had done myself. I'd been the rogue of the family on occasions but he was loyal to the end. In the quiet of the night, negative feelings would creep into my mind now and then. There were times that I thought of myself 'as the disease' and there were times when my RA defined the person I was. *RA was me, I was RA. I was my disease, my disease was me.* When I was in my twenties it was all my friends and family ever asked about. In some ways it was like identity theft. RA had robbed me of my own identity; my sense of self. Disease does that. Perhaps this was because I was diagnosed so young, or maybe it was because I had surrendered to my RA in the past. I don't really know. But I became: 'Karen Ager, she's the one with arthritis'.

The disease became synonymous with my name—like 'she's tall'. Somehow this sort of truism is acceptable with diseases—he's got cancer, she's got MS, he's got Parkinson's, she's in a wheelchair. It is not politically correct to define someone by their skin or their nationality so I wondered why it was okay to define by illness. In New York I felt I was finding 'me' for the first time since my diagnosis. No-one knew—except Charlotte—and that was refreshing. At home people were starting to say 'she's living in New York'', rather than 'she's got arthritis, that old people's disease'.

I also felt in some strange, even perverse way that RA had given me a voice in the family. Steve was the pilot and I got attention through my disease. RA was my alter ego. It had become a metaphor for me. I loved my brother because he had never thought of me in this way. To him, I was simply his sister, Kaz, whom he loved and of whom he was proud. But this was Steve all over. He'd never been any different. Ever since I can remember, he was keen to be around his sister, full of pride and playing Mr Positive. His teenage Aussie Rules trophy for Best Team Player was proof of that.

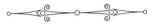

Cosmopolitans and margaritas filled the rest of my summer days. American men, even strangers, are known for their generosity. Most of the time when I was out with my girlfriends men would send over drinks for us. It's a 'cultural thing' and it's rude to decline the gesture. It worked for me because money was tight, New York was expensive and my wage was $10,000 less than what I had been earning in Oz, but somehow I made do.

During the school year I had taken a job as a hostess at a midtown (or shit town as I sometimes call this part of the city) bar on Friday nights to help make ends meet. But standing all night wrecked me for the entire weekend. My ankle joints throbbed badly after my shift and I'd hobble home, close the curtains and not face the world again until Monday morning. There seemed to be no point being in New York, but Gotham had a hold on me. I wanted to stay at all costs.

During the North American summer I spent my time with other Australian expat friends who had become like family to me. My Aussie girlfriends kept their collective fingers on the hot button of reality and didn't hesitate to challenge me about my choice to be single. They suggested I had fears about intimacy. Perhaps this was true. I'd been hurt so much in the past, they said, that maybe I was scared to love again. I didn't really agree. It was more about a self-inflicted isolation because of my disease. Being single was easier than sharing the burden of my secret in a new relationship.

I could see how transient New York was and how difficult it can be to make friends. People move to Gotham and often leave after a year or two. This is what happened with Kelly Longley, the then wife of ex-Australian Olympic basketball player and Chicago Bulls/ New York Knicks player, Luc Longley. Kelly was stunning. She was a six-foot-tall blonde American gal who had been displaced so many times because of Luc's basketball career that she was like a foreigner in NY. Kelly and I hit it off at the Australia Day Ball, a black tie event run by the American Australian Association. A week or so later, I spent Super Bowl with them at a party at their place in Connecticut. Kelly and I liked to party together. Another night I was picked up by their driver; which, by the way, was a concept foreign to me. 'Having a driver' was as 'New York' as Central Park. They whisked me away to an award night for the US restaurant industry with Kelly. Dubbed 'The Oscars of the food and beverage industry' by the *NY Times*, I frocked up for the James Beard Awards. Kelly and their manager (minus husband Luc who, at the last minute, had basketball playoff commitments) welcomed me with a glass of Moet as they picked me up. Never completely at home in this situation, I went to get out of the SUV and smashed the bottle of Moet on the ground as it *and I* rolled out of the car. A few months later, Luc and Kelly moved to Western Australia—Luc's home territory—and I never heard from them again. But that's the nature of the beast in New York. Losing friends is part of the equation.

The 'Moet incident' reminded me of my Dad all over. I always looked the part but my lack of coordination often made me unravel. dad was much the same—at times he had no social graces, much like Peter Sellers at *The Party*.

When I visited some other new friends in Connecticut and they were showing me around their home I made the comment: 'That's a nice trophy.' I didn't have a clue at the time that it was an Emmy. This was typical Kaz.

Chapter 14
Comfortably Numb

R eality check: you have an incurable disease. Had I forgotten or was I still in partial denial? Sometimes it was easier to just ignore the truth. I'd become a master at hiding my arthritis over the last 20 years. Couple this with 'looking well' and being in New York where only Charlotte knew about my RA and before I knew it I was fooling myself back into believing and behaving as if there was nothing wrong. I had late nights and drank as much as I pleased and acted as if I were like the rest of the party girls. But there was a big difference; most of them were probably medication free and were 'allowed' to drink. I self-soothed by alcohol. New York had given me the ticket I needed to slip partially back into denial. It was at my own peril.

My suitcase was full of medicine—dozens of prescription bottles stashed with my belongings—and easy access to my medication throughout the year hadn't helped either. I tossed medications into my mouth morning and night as if it was the normal thing to do. I was so matter of fact about it that I didn't think twice. As long as I was getting through my school days and was able to go out on the weekend I didn't care about what the meds were doing to my body. I knew I had to be on the drugs, I accepted that much. But I didn't take any responsibility for being sick. I didn't seek out a doctor in New York until my meds were nearly finished, which was months after I arrived. Even when I got my medical cover partially paid by work, I just kept swallowing my pills without consultation. I didn't do any research about the side effects of the medications, or go for my blood tests—though I knew I should have been doing this. I didn't care about tomorrow.

In a letter of introduction from my rheumatologist in Australia to the doctor who would be treating me in New York he wrote:

> *I saw Karen for review and was disturbed, but not terribly surprised to find that her last blood count was 5 months ago. This is fairly hazardous while on a drug like Imuran. It is not infrequently a challenge to have Karen undertake her regular appropriate blood testing.*

Mentally I had come a long way towards accepting the disease— but I still had a long way to go. At least I'd stopped blaming Mum for my RA and the way I felt about it. That was good. And I'd stopped blaming myself for not being a good enough daughter and that somehow my disease was my penance. That was good. But I knew I wasn't healed yet, actually I wasn't even close. I was still bargaining for freedom from the responsibility of it. My reckless, self-destructive ways of behaving was a symptom of that.

On another level, however, I was bargaining for a morsel of control. It was my body, so I wanted it to be my decision whether to have blood tests or not. I felt I couldn't influence much else about the disease. I was tired of relying on doctors' time, opinion and knowledge to do a good job. They often seemed to end up taking control and then, as the 'sick person' I was left ringside while the doctor and the disease battle it out for supremacy.

Also there was that constant feeling of being bullied by my arthritis. It was always lurking in the background, threatening to wreck New York for me and take my lifestyle away. The perceived 'bully' element intimidated me in a similar way to when I was a kid in primary school. I had big ears which poked out through my string-blonde page-boy hairstyle. If my brother wasn't in the school playground to protect me I would get teased and called 'big ears'. Sometimes the other kids would even steal my lunch money right out of my hands while I was waiting in line. That's what bullies do. They choose your most vulnerable time then ambush to inflict maximum emotional and physical pain. RA does the same. I constantly flared right before a big event at school, a special date or the 24-hour flight home from New York to Australia.

My flares were becoming more frequent as my body became less responsive to the meds and I began to develop a deep fear of the pain that came with each joint eruption. It was an exhausting way to live, or shall I say exist. I couldn't stop the cycle. I had never taken the time to think about it all and 'break my fear apart' so I *couldn't* stop the cycle. My stretch in New York had distracted me from learning about myself and my arthritis; I think I had designed it that way. Geographical changes tend to do that. They mask the problem for a while, just like cortisone shots to the joints, then the problem usually comes back with a vengeance.

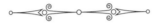

It was the second week of July 2001. By now I had been in New York City for 11 months and had survived my first winter and school year. Shuffling through the snow had stiffened my ankles. Bending and reaching, sitting and standing—doing all that I needed to do to get my six-foot frame aligned with my three-foot-tall students—had almost become too painful to manage in the end. The last couple of months of school I had trouble holding a pen to correct the kids' work and writing on the whiteboard because of my shoulders. I knew it was time to listen to my body.

My supply of medications was about to dry up. This didn't really matter since my arsenal had been no match for the wicked flare-ups I suffered that first winter and it had been months since I felt like my disease was under control. It was becoming so brutally painful that I could feel it in my bones, literally. I think I had become an idle bystander, encouraging more joint destruction through my own inaction. My disease had permission to run amok. But I was no innocent bystander anymore, I was as guilty as the bully; as guilty as the kid who stands by and says nothing.

I made an appointment with a rheumatologist. I pushed the buzzer of her Park Avenue suite feeling very nervous about my prognosis. The doctor's office looked more like a lounge-room to me. Red velvet chairs with gold side studs were positioned around the room for easy access and antique framed pictures decorated the walls.

I silently waited. I dared not look at the crooked fingers of the elderly people in the room—a future that included similar disfigurements scared me.

The doctor who called me into her office was an elegant, well-dressed woman. She had the stature of a ballerina with the beauty and looks of a classic black-and-white film star. Not more than 45 years old, her high-heeled patent leather shoes caught the light of the chandelier in her consulting room. She was gentle and calming in manner. I could tell she wanted to help— she knew I was in a lot of pain. After running her fingers soothingly over every joint in my body, Dr Marchetta delivered her diagnosis.

'Your disease is very aggressive, Karen. In 20 years you will be severely debilitated, there's no doubt about that, maybe even in a wheelchair.'

She let these words sink in before continuing.

'But you do have some choices.'

She went on to tell me that I could continue with my pills and watch my health decline or try a new biological medicine that could do more than just slow RA's progress and blunt its pain.

'These biologics might actually stop further damage by blocking the destructive protein RA patients like you overproduce,' she explained.

My eyes widened as I embraced the thought of something that, to me, sounded almost like a cure. Her charming voice went on.

'One of the new drugs is a breakthrough biological medication called Remicade. It has a biological agent that is given intravenously in the doctor's rooms.'

Dr Marchetta told me that the treatments were called 'infusions' and that the medication came with warnings of possible side effects ranging from infection to kidney damage and on to heart failure.

I had already 'lost' my right shoulder, hip, hand, knees and feet to this illness. As tears welled up in my eyes I could see that even though I'd accepted this damn disease I was still carrying the burden of it heavily in my heart. I'd lost all expectations of ever feeling any better, or ever finding a cure. I had accepted having pain with every footstep, of not being able to raise my arm over my head, of struggling to turn a key in a lock and of feeling exhausted most of the time. I thought about why I was single. I was beginning to grasp that it was not just because I was scared about getting hurt again; it was also that I didn't want to burden anyone else with my illness. My disease had dictated my world and I was prepared to be alone forever and forgo being loved or having a child because I didn't want someone else to have to accept and share my burden.

I was alone in America. I could barely manage the job that had brought me here. Was this a golden opportunity for me—Remicade was not yet available in Australia—or a fast track to debilitating and possibly fatal, battles with RA?

My answers arrived when I left the doctor's surgery.

As I came out of the office I noticed a blind man walking down Park Avenue. The man was tapping his white stick as he shuffled between city workers and lunchtime pedestrians trying to avoid a construction site. Yellow and black caution tape was wrapped around a web of wooden stakes and orange mesh temporary fencing surrounding a gaping hole in the sidewalk. Suddenly his cane got tangled in the netting. He tumbled over his feet, losing his balance and falling awkwardly on to the uneven ground. Without hesitation, or even an appeal for help he brushed himself off, stood up and kept going. He faced his fears every moment of every day.

I arrived home and made an appointment for an infusion.

It was time to face my fears.

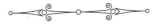

I was on my way to my first treatment. As I walked down 2nd Avenue past East 34th Street I was awestruck by the Empire State dwarfing the surrounding buildings. Its antenna pierced through the clouds and it looked like a dark citadel where a powerful wizard resided. It was a surreal image. Now it was a backdrop to my trip down the Yellow Brick Road as I slowly limped, rather than skipped, towards my magician who would hopefully provide an answer to my biggest wish.

As I entered the clinic I felt optimistic for the first time in years. The waiting room was thick with body smells. I found a chair in the corner and hoped no-one would sit next to me. I sat quietly thinking about the wait I'd had to get to this moment—to have hope again. It seemed like a lifetime ago that I was a teenager on the beach in Black Rock anchored to my towel by my hip. It had been a long road through the 1980s and 90s without a medical breakthrough like the new biological drug my body was about to trial. Some people wait 20 years to find that special person, others wait a lifetime to bear a child. I had waited for this. The promise of better health excited me but I was scared too. The adverse side effects worried me but not as much as a life with debilitating pain which dominated my every thought and movement. I nervously flicked through the pages of a ruffled magazine until I heard my name called: 'Karen Ager.'

'That's me,' I answered as I tried to get my aching body out of my seat without looking like the tin man in the *Wizard of Oz*. As I followed the nurse to the infusion room I said a silent prayer: 'God, I need your help. Please make this work, I need this to work.'

My right arm was swabbed clean with an alcohol wipe and a tourniquet applied. A few taps on my vein and it rose on command to the surface of the skin. The cold syringe was inserted like a sewing needle catching the threads of an uneven hem. At one end of the needle was a valve which was capped closed while the medication was prepared. The little black rubber wheels on the silver IV pole squeaked loudly as the matronly African-American nurse dragged it beside my chair. I didn't tell her that this was my first dose of Remicade infusion. I don't think it would have made a difference. A square plastic bag of clear medication hung off the hook. The lines from my vein to the drip were uncapped and inserted into each other without a drop of blood escaping. As I watched each trickle of Remicade flow along the clear plastic tube and into my body I felt desperately alone.

One voice in my head played out the 'poor me' role. 'You're going through this all by yourself on the other side of the world without the support of family.'

But another voice whispered an antidote.

'You'll be fine. You can do this. You have support if you need it. Just get on with it and stop feeling sorry for yourself.'

The voices were thrashing it out in my head as I sat and waited for any adverse reactions to the drug. The nurse checked the IV every few minutes and I watched each drop fall from the bag into the long tube.

I knew the first 15 minutes of the infusion were critical. Time would soon tell whether my body would reject the drug. A red rash, swollen lips, shortness of breath or low blood pressure would be the first telltale signs.

I'd made it to the tenth minute of the infusion and I felt fine. Half an hour went slowly by and I still felt good. The voices in my head became subdued. Somehow I had rallied my spiritual energy, focusing on everyone I loved and thinking about how happy we would all feel if this worked for me. As the medication continued to be dribbled into my body I felt more and more confident.

'Stop being so scared. Picture yourself getting better. Every drop will fight off whatever is bad in my blood and soon I'll feel better.' The voices in my head encouraged me.

Two hours later it was all over. The IV was removed by a swift tug of the needle, pressure applied and I was free to go. I'd be back in two weeks to complete my 'initiation' and then the maintenance stage would kick in with a treatment every six to eight weeks.

The only way out of the treatment building was past the 'Please pay here' window. A large lady behind the counter said in a gruff voice: 'That's $20.'

I handed over a crumpled greenback and left. It was a good deal. My health insurance had approved the treatment before my infusion so the cost was nothing for me to worry about; I was covered. I had paid the high premium for US health insurance for a year and it had been worth it. If I had not had health insurance the cost of each treatment would have been US$4000.

When I woke the next day I was almost pain-free. I had not felt like this in years. It was a gift from God. I couldn't imagine that walking could be so easy. I think I felt normal. I began to notice that I was able to do things without thinking twice about whether I could manage or not. I could pass a plate without carefully considering the way I needed to hold it. I could walk up and down stairs without tackling each step one at a time. I could pull the duvet cover up over my shoulders without pain. When I reached over to plug something in to a power point I was able to bend down and 'just do it'. All this and it was just the morning after the treatment!

In my secret heart I knew that I was damaged goods, but maybe now I could allow someone to love me, even if I had this crippling disease because there was hope.

I was crying when I called my mum.

'I can walk properly. There's no pain, Mum, there's no pain.'

Sobbing into the telephone she said: 'I'm so proud of you darling.'

It seemed like the RA medications available to me in the United States had taken a quantum leap. I was hopeful that I'd be boosted out of my never-ending cycle of periods of relative good health and then disastrous flares that sent me into abysmal pain and, quite often, hospital beds.

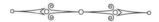

I've thought a lot about my first IV infusion; about the isolation of disease and the loneliness of the moment when the sickly green curtain is pulled across and you're shut out from the rest of the world. It's a moment of no control; when there's not much choice anymore, just a road map of what you have to do and a landscape of obstacles to overcome. As I get further into my 40s I know better that we all have crosses to bear. I've tried to talk about feelings of isolation with my friends, male and female, who have had their own health struggles with AIDs, MS, RA and ovarian cancer. In most cases the pain of it all is too much for them to talk about and they further separate themselves from their disease because they don't want to be pitied. I wondered how they coped with their 'green curtain moment'.

A friend with MS said: 'Only last week I was sitting in the doctor's office waiting to see my new doctor. There were many people in wheelchairs and it was very frightening. There are always moments in your life when you're totally alone and the isolation can be overwhelming. At those times I try to look deep into myself and think about the people I love. As I sat in the office waiting, very aware of that loneliness, a song came on the radio called 'I'll be Watching You' by Sting. Many years ago on my first overseas trip that song was a hit and my mother and I said that it would be 'our song'. I shed a tear and knew that I was not alone and everything would be okay. It's the love of the special people in our lives that keeps us strong and optimistic.' In a strange quirk of fate this friend, and now ally, was Venessa. She had bravely faced the shock of her own autoimmune disease diagnoses in recent years and somehow already had the wisdom to be thankful for all that her MS had taught her about relationships and about herself.

Another friend who had cervical cancer wrote: 'I think I would like to have tea with the interior decorator who won the contract to choose the decor for the hospital I'm in. I'd make him or her sit in this corridor, on this poxy vinyl chair, behind this green curtain, drinking this vile concoction, waiting to be laid out and injected with dye for a scan to determine if the past three months of chemo and radiology has worked. Or not! It's like getting a permission slip for the next three months of my life: "Here you go, Mrs Scott-Handley. All looks clear so come back and see us in three months for your next check."

'I could scream out loud with this whole pathetic scene right now if it would make the ache in my stomach and the lump in my throat disappear. I've told myself so many times this morning to just shut up. Stop doing this to the point where the mental angst has become a physical pain in my gut. I made up the most dismal excuses to be here on my own. I even yelled at my husband so that he wouldn't take the morning off work to sit here and witness this. I don't want a single soul to see what cancer has reduced me to. From the time I was diagnosed with cervical cancer through to having a *radical* hysterectomy (as opposed to your run-of-the-mill, stay-at-home, mum-type normal one) I had an army of support carrying me on.

'My closest girlfriends became my therapy circle—they listened to my rantings via email and lived through my being diagnosed with the most unfashionable disease on the planet. There's no major fashion houses knocking out charity T-shirts with pink ribbons for this one.

They told me I looked great, even when I resembled a puffer fish from the drugs I had to take and made sure that my husband—my lovely, darling husband who moved hemispheres to marry me—always had a scaffolding of good friends around him.

'But I can't bring myself to explain to them how alone and insignificant I feel in my world right now—surrounded by some dullard's pissed-up attempts at creating an environment that supposedly helps people heal.

'I just don't want them to know about the train wreck that has been left behind now that the surgery and chemo and laser blasting has finished. I survived. I'm lucky and has it made me view the world any differently? I want to talk about something else. Anything else but cancer. I don't want people hanging around me, feeling useless and lost for words. Making light conversation that just echoes off the dull walls, highlighting just how empty and useless this entire scene is. To the outside world I'm back to the old me—loud, opinionated, energetic. I don't want them to resort to pity—that "head cocked to the side" look we save for old people.'

I knew from my own struggle with RA and my despair that the isolation of disease changes your soul. I didn't want to listen to the 'poor me' talk either, nor feel pity for my friends. We're not 'poor anything'; we're empowered because of disease and somehow, after all is said and done, enriched by our struggles.

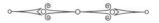

A few days after my infusion, I boarded the flying kangaroo, bound for Oz. I needed to see my family and get some perspective back into my life. Reconnecting with home was essential to my survival in New York. I began to sweat before I found my seat on the Qantas 747, anxious at the thought of trying to lift my bag into the allocated locker while the line of people backed up behind me. I expected the usual brawl with my luggage because of my sore wrists, elbows and shoulders. It was like being a college wrestler trying to get my bag into a submissive position. Over the years I'd worked out a technique, lift my 'carry-on' halfway, cradle it in one arm, then elevate it just enough to reach the edge of the overhead compartment and push the bag the rest of the way in with my head and a good hand if I had one. This flight was different. I snapped open the overhead bin easily and lifted my bag up in one smooth graceful motion. No-one huffed and puffed impatiently behind me and I didn't have a hundred eyes on me watching the struggle.

Three hundred kilometres (186 miles) out of Sydney and my body did not feel as wrecked as I had expected from the 27-hour commute. My feet were swollen but they were not painful and I did not have any new hot spots to work around. My body had handled the flight beautifully. The benefits of my new drug were broader than I'd ever imagined.

A great feeling of pride in Australia swept over me as I gazed out the window across the wing tip towards the country I loved. As we descended over Sydney's magical beaches and glistening harbour a teardrop ran down my check. I was home. The morning sun had risen casting its winter rays over a cloudless baby-blue sky. Seeing Australia's rocky coastline forced me to think about Captain Cook's journey and navigation along unchartered waters. His expedition to claim Australia for the British along such a dramatically rugged shoreline seemed unimaginable. My stomach fluttered. I couldn't wait to see my family.

I love the Aussie manner—'fair dinkum', easy going and positive. Our confident, capable attitude is bred from our struggles with the harsh elements of our land. We're resilient in the face of crises, tell it like it is and shorten or twist each other's names to show affection. Barry becomes Bazza, John—Johnno, Sharon—Shazza, Kerry—Kez.

I overheard one of the American passengers ask an Aussie on board: 'What do you do for fun here?'

He replied: 'Well, mate we go to the beach, fish, have a bet on the horses and a beer at the pub.'

After almost a year in New York I needed to spend some serious time in the bush. Having nature all around helps me to relax. It's calming. I arranged to meet my dad in Broome. Broome is rich in Aboriginal culture and lies 2000 km (1242 miles) up the coast from

Perth in Western Australia. It was once known as the Queen City of the North because of its pearling trade. It has a vibrant history of rebuilding itself in tough economic times, especially after it was attacked by the Japanese in 1942—when most of the residents fled. Today it has a population of more than 10,000. Cable Beach, which is not far from what the locals call 'town' is a 22-km (13-mile) stretch of sand, red stone cliffs and turquoise water. In the late 1880s the main means of telecommunications between Broome and Indonesia was a submarine telegraph cable which linked the town with the rest of the world and communicated pearl prices as they swung around in ebbs and flows as much as Wall Street stocks do today.

New York seemed like a million miles away as I sat on Cable Beach watching the sunset unfold before my eyes. Red, yellow, pink and orange splashed across the sky and over the turquoise water of the Indian Ocean with such perfection that it could have been a canvas. I was lost in my own thoughts about the natural beauty of what I was seeing until I became distracted by a group of six Aboriginal boys. Running along the sand their shadows formed perfect silhouettes of athleticism as they bounced an Aussie Rules football and kicked it to one another. Their muscular bodies leapt effortlessly to great heights to catch the ball. In the distance were two lone surfers riding some easy waves in an ocean which they could have called their own. A solitary fisherman stood on the water's edge hoping for a nibble on the end of his line.

As I left Cable Beach I heard three men, all about 65 years of age, having a conversation.

One asked: 'How long will we be here?

His mate answered: 'It depends on the scenery.'

I knew he meant the women and not the sunset I had just been admiring, but I loved his ageless Aussie spirit.

A few days together were all that dad and I needed to reconnect. He was easy to be with and, as always, quiet most of the time, accidentally funny and surprisingly philosophical. He loved to chat to the Aboriginal people. When I was growing up, one of dad's best mates was an Aborigine called Snowy Barnes, who lived in a remote and dusty gold mining town called Leonora. Snowy was enchanted by dad's metal detector and together they would go prospecting for gold and study geological maps to stake out claims of land in search of the elusive golden nugget. The relationship worked. The telephone would ring in the Black Rock house and we all knew to accept the reverse charge call from Snowy who would soon get on the line with his deeply accented Aboriginal English, which sounded almost cockney to me.

The holiday with dad raced by, as did the week or two I spent travelling up and down the east coast spending time with Mum and Steve. All of my family and friends expressed the same feelings of joy that I was doing so well in Manhattan. While part of it was the Remicade in my veins, they could also see that I was content with my life in New York. When the time came for me to say goodbye it was easier for all of us because my move had worked out so well for me.

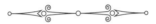

As I slipped my keys into my new 'shoebox' apartment I thought about how good it felt to be back in Gotham. I had quickly moved apartments just before my trip home. It was another compact living space in the same building, but it was $200 a month cheaper and on a corner. It looked characterless without furniture but because I was now on the permanent staff at work they had offered to ship my personal things from Oz. There would be a six-week wait. I slept on my futon and figured the time would pass quickly until my bed, couch and linen arrived. It was time to call Manhattan home.

Being pain-free had put me on a permanent high. The warm September sun brought out the best in New Yorkers and when tennis champion Lleyton Hewitt won the US Open, Aussies banded together to celebrate. After a day sweating it out at the US Open my girlfriend and I partied with Lleyton and other expats at a Park Avenue sports bar. It was a 'New York moment' as they say. Everything felt right about being back in my new 'home'. But two days after Hewitt's win the world changed forever.

Chapter 15
A Brave New World

The terrorist attack on the World Trade Center on 11 September 2001 speared through my heart. Isolated and petrified by the events that had taken place, I turned to my journal.

> *11 September:* Today—9/11—was the saddest day of my life. I don't know how I even feel or how to describe it. There's sadness everywhere. It's devastating; an overwhelming force of negativity. There's so much trepidation in the city, horror on faces and fear about what might happen next. I just feel so heartbroken for the children who are waiting for mummy or daddy to come home. Is it selfish to say I am scared and lonely? I need my family. My friends have husbands to lean on.
>
> We stand united in this tragedy but are so wounded by it. As I write this they say more than 200 firemen have lost their lives. I sit here staring on to First Avenue opposite a desolate United Nations. I am numb, unable to write about how I really feel. I am just so worried about the kids in my care.
>
> God bless us all.

'Darling, are you okay? I've seen it on the news. What about the kids?' Mum said frantically without a breath, interrupting my lesson.

'Mum, I can't talk now. I've got to get back to the children. We're fine.'

'I love you, Kaz.'

'I love you too, Mum.'

I put down the phone, sucked in some air and returned to 'my kids' as if nothing was wrong.

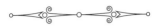

Sitting on a purple-cushioned chair in my Grade Two classroom with the morning sun warming the room, I looked at the innocent expressions of the children as I called the roll. The bright faces of the seven-year-olds assigned to me for the year are children of every skin tone, from many cultures and traditions, who eat different kinds of food, listen to different styles of music, hear different stories and celebrate the holidays of many religions. My mind strayed. How could this tragedy have happened today with so much hope for world peace in one room?

It was only the second week of the school year. I was in charge of 20 children whose names I was only just learning. I didn't know their idiosyncrasies and we weren't emotionally connected yet. Today nothing else mattered but them. I wouldn't tell my new little friends what had happened in New York a few miles down the road; their parents had to do that. My job was to keep them safe and to try to be calm myself so that they wouldn't pick up on my anxiety.

Ice-creams did the trick. Strolling through the hallway with a trolley of vanilla ice-cream cups and chocolate chip cookies came the school's male secretary, Mr Stackman. A tall masculine guy in his thirties, he commanded respect because of his physical presence and deep voice. He looked out of place behind a stewardess-style cart.

The treats were given because it was the start of the school year— or so we said. The kids slurped and licked their lips, ignorant of the mayhem happening in Manhattan. My classroom routine continued as normal until parents arrived to pick up their children throughout the day. The school was a sanctuary. It was calm, almost peaceful.

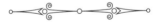

A few hours after the September 11 attacks parents who worked in lower Manhattan began to arrive to pick up their children. Those who lived near the Twin Towers stocked up on essential items and then set out for the 5-km (3-mile) hike along the East River to 23rd Street where the school sits on prime real estate.

The children wriggled and sat cross-legged on the carpet as I read them *Wilfrid Gordon McDonald Partridge*—a wonderful Australian children's book written by Mem Fox and illustrated by Julie Vivas. Twitching, picking their noses and fiddling with scraps of paper on the floor I imagined they had the same fidgety energy as Wilfrid Gordon, the little boy in the story who was trying to help his 96-year-old friend 'find' her memory.

We had got to the part in the story where Wilfrid, who was always asking questions, called on a Mr Tippet who was crazy about cricket and asked: 'What's a memory?'

The answer was: 'Something that makes you cry my boy, something that makes you cry.'

Although these children didn't know it as I read the words in the story, *I* understood that the memory of this day would probably always be 'something that makes them cry'. I silently wondered how they would recall September 11, 2001 in the future and what would spark their emotions. Would it be the story about Wilfrid Gordon, the smell of a chocolate chip cookie or perhaps the taste of vanilla ice-cream? I knew that right now I had to be the best teacher I could be and as calm as I could be, for the sake of their emotional future.

The children sat facing the East River, their backs to the doorway. As I continued to read to them in a gentle tone I became distracted by a Singaporian father entering the classroom. He wore a white, tie-less business shirt and suit pants which were both covered with dust. His black shoes bore the same light, sandy-hued film. I knew he worked near the Twin Towers. Our eyes locked, sharing our fear.

'Can I take Sophie now?' he said quietly as he motioned to her to come.

Their bodies joined in a bear hug as he stroked her shoulder-length hair and rubbed her back. As father and daughter left the classroom our eyes met again.

'Thank you, Miss Ager, thank you,' he whispered with a sigh of relief and strained half smile.

I also shared September 11 with my colleagues, Charlotte and Venessa. Charlotte was taking care of her class across the corridor. Her high hopes for a stress-free new school year after the loss of her parents were shattered. She left school with a colleague frantically trying to locate her girlfriend's husband. Venessa and Al lived in the heart of the destruction. I was now the teacher of their youngest daughter. There was no way I was going anywhere until I could safely hand her over to them. They arrived at school in the early afternoon having run all the way from lower Manhattan to collect their three children from school. I saw strength and courage in them as a couple that day. They were bonded in their distress and in their need to protect their children. I saw love.

It was mid-afternoon when I finally left work. I walked home in silence with my Japanese teaching assistant, Kimiko. We headed north towards 34th Street along the East River. The beautiful weather and serenity of the waterway did not match the events of the day. On our right, bobbing along the river one after the other were New York ferries. As they docked at the midtown mooring on this cloudless September day I caught a glimpse of nearby NYU (New York University) Hospital. Doctors stood anxiously next to lines of empty trolleys waiting for victims to treat. But there were none. The casualties they had hoped for were not making it out of The Towers alive. Even though Kimiko and I didn't talk much on that walk we needed each other. She was single too and had to face the world feeling as unprotected as I did. We both understood that. Nothing had to be said. As we walked by the ferry terminal, a mirage of dazed and frightened expressions flashed into our path. Stony eyes fixed on us. Faces were scratched and white with dust. Designer suits were ripped, men were without jackets and women were shoeless. High heels had been cast aside as New Yorkers headed for the bridges and the safety of Queens and Brooklyn. It was like we were all refugees fleeing from an occupied city.

We were stopped by a rumpled stranger wearing jeans and a torn T-shirt. He was choking on his tears and running on adrenaline and sweat poured off his brow as he stood in the street shaking and saying,

'I have the Twin Towers falling down on video.'

Before we knew it the camera was shoved in our faces. Fear and human instinct for survival united us, but there were no words to explain how I felt when I saw the footage of The Towers falling for the first time. School had been a sanctuary for me as well as the kids. Facing the real world on September 11 was not something I wanted to do.

We kept on walking in silence. Crying, Kimiko and I hugged each other as we said goodbye.

'Call me if you need to,' I said as we went our separate ways, each with fear in our eyes. I watched her back disappear into the distance as she walked away from me on 42nd Street.

As I walked inside my apartment I stopped for a moment and tried to make sense of this terror and the craziness. I couldn't. I felt completely and utterly lost. Three footsteps into my apartment and I could see the red light was flashing furiously on my telephone message machine. I pressed play.

First message:

'Hi Karen, it's Dani. I am in New York as you know. We had a good time for Lachlan's birthday. I am shopping downtown today. I will call you later to arrange a catch up.' She'd left the message before the aircraft hit the Twin Towers.

Tearful messages were left from Australian friends who didn't know the geography of New York and who feared for my safety, but I couldn't focus on what they were saying because all I kept hearing was: 'I'm shopping downtown.'

Dani was the parent of a gorgeous Grade One girl I had taught in Sydney. She and her husband were in New York for Lachlan Murdoch's 30th birthday. I tried to call Australia and her hotel, but my telephone didn't work and I had not been able to afford a cell phone. My body sank awkwardly down my 'living room' wall. I sat on the floor unable to find the energy to move, staring blankly at the walls of my apartment. I wanted to run. I loved my job but living in terror, in a rundown apartment without furniture, left me wondering why I was so far from Australia; living in a city that was under threat.

Six floors up and adjacent to the United Nations I stood at my window watching 14-wheeler Department of Sanitation trucks heaped with road salt form an impenetrable fortress of rubber and steel. An army of police and soldiers ordered them into defensive position as if they were a battalion of tanks. Their engines roared like beasts as they were herded to their location before the brakes screeched and the engines were cut. Choppers circled the night sky as if it was a war zone and paired members of the SWAT team guarded every corner of the UN building. Looking down on the street to First Avenue I couldn't hear the usual hustle and bustle of traffic heading uptown, or honking car horns. Once the defences had been set and people were with their loved ones, the city was eerily quiet as everyone waited for what would happen next.

New York, the city that never sleeps, was mostly deserted.

An hour or so later I ventured out. I walked past the Tudor City gardens, crossed 2nd Avenue looking south towards downtown. New York was clad in a haze of dusty clouds. The mood in the city was much darker than the ash that was settling on everything around me. All was still silent except for the sirens. I was headed for the nearest public telephone box so I could call home; my phone had no dial tone. I found one on East 43rd Street—a dark and dingy side street which housed the backside of Pfizer headquarters and reflected my mood. I hid in the hood of the silver booth as if it were able to shield me from another violent attack. Already posted on every spare side were flyers with the faces of beautiful young men and women smiling at me.

'MISSING, MISSING, MISSING, MISSING'…

The words shouted at me over and over and over again.

'MISSING, MISSING, MISSING'.

I sobbed into the phone.

'Mum, they're not coming home. These people are just not coming home.'

I could not face being alone that night so I went to an Aussie girlfriend's apartment right opposite the ferry mooring and NYU Hospital where I'd watched the doctors wheeling in empty trolleys a few hours before. Together we made it through the night with the help of a few glasses of wine.

School was closed on 12 September. I was in a confused state of mind as I walked through mid-town Manhattan in search of the

Sofitel Hotel. I was scared; jumping with fright every time a bus went over a pot hole and made a thunderous noise. Dani, my friend who'd been shopping downtown on September 11, was staying there with her husband. Many phone lines on Manhattan Island were not working because of heavy damage to the telecommunications buildings adjacent to the World Trade Center. I hadn't been able to contact Dani, so I anxiously scuttled along 42nd street towards Fifth Avenue.

As I walked across town, sirens, like an unknown animal wailing, drowned out my footsteps. Red lights, blue lights, yellow lights and white lights blinked at me and demanded my attention. I couldn't focus on where I was going. Swarms of people gathered outside buildings in response to calls to evacuate. Others scurried back inside after yet another false alarm.

After getting lost on familiar streets I knocked on Dani's hotel room door, saying out loud: 'God, please let her be there; please let her be there.'

A split second later Dani answered my knock, leaning in towards the door so that her body was half-hidden.

'I needed to know if you were okay,' I said as we stooped inwards to hug each other.

'I'm all right, are you?' she whispered gently in my ear as she pulled her body away.

'I think so.'

Her face was soft and make up free as she stood amidst a backdrop of afternoon sunshine beaming through curtained windows. Her blonde hair was shining in the shafts of patterned light as the sunrays fell to the floor.

'Where's Carlo?' I asked with trepidation.

She answered in one long sentence without stopping for air,

'He's at a meeting, he's fine…do you want to get a drink?'

The Gaby Bar at the hotel was far enough for us to venture. Elegant French décor surrounded the glass-top circular bar. Dani and I sat down on the high-backed leather stools and ordered a bottle of cabernet. Jason the bartender was polishing fingerprints off long-stemmed flutes while deep in thought. Four shelves of spirits stacked up behind him as the SKYY vodka bottles cast a blue hue on their platforms. It suddenly struck me that we were not alone at the bar, even though it was only 3.30 in the afternoon. Many New Yorkers were drinking rocket fuel. It was obvious why.

We sat at the bar and talked. Dani second-guessed herself about her decision to come to New York , leaving her kids in Australia. I told her she was being too hard on herself. Deep inside she knew that. She could never have anticipated what had happened the day before. I shared secrets with her I'd kept about my health for the three years I'd known her. The destruction of the Twin Towers had numbed me and driven away my fears about people's opinions. I didn't care anymore. The horrors of 'that day' also liberated me to say 'I love you' to family and friends. Dani was there for me to lean on. We both needed to feel close to one another because of what we'd been through. It was as complex and as simple as that.

I used her cell phone to call Australia and to check on Charlotte. Sara O'Hare joined us later for a drink. I declined an invitation to dine with Dani and the Murdochs. My world had changed and so had my values.

I needed to be home safely and in touch with my family.

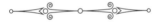

The events in New York that day forced me to think about love. That may sound strange but, as well as the pain and trauma, it was a wake-up call. My family's love for me shone through as they collectively decided dad needed to fly over to New York to help me through the days and weeks after the attacks. Once he arrived we went to Ground Zero to pay our respects. The World Trade Center was still smoldering. The air was thick. Our hearts were heavy. The energy was overwhelming. It was so powerfully sad and depressing that being silent was the most respectful thing to do. I needed dad's support and he was there. Friends repeatedly tried to contact me from all over the world as a show of their affection. But perhaps the most unforgettable sign of love was from the parents of the kids I taught. There was no warning, no build up to the unspeakable happening.

When these mothers and fathers sent their children to school they kissed them goodbye and trusted me with their most precious thing in the world. I deeply respected that faith and in return I got their love and I saw their love for their children. After suffering through the trauma of the attacks and fearing for their own lives, all that mattered was being reunited with their children. As I watched father and son and mother and daughter come together again, I became a spectator in the classroom and gained a new appreciation for the love of a parent for their child. The Class of 01/02 will always be precious to me.

The Aussie expats stuck together at this time and met about a week or so later for a candlelight vigil in midtown. It was the first time many of us had ventured out. Hugs and stiff smiles replaced words that night. On Friday 28 September 2001 at 10.00 a.m. the Australian and New Zealand Consulates had an interfaith Memorial Prayer Service at the Epiphany Church right by my school. The Australian Minister for Foreign Affairs, Alexander Downer, was there along with the Consul Generals from each country. The Australian, New Zealand and American national anthems were sung by a choir led by soloists Lana Cantrell and Simon O'Neill to a silent congregation of tearful expats.

I stood at the back of the church unable to find a place on a pew because of the crowds of mourners who were there from all denominations. I bowed my head trying to muffle sobs as I listened to prayers for compassion, in what now seemed like a dangerous and frightening world. Voices singing 'The Prayer of St. Francis', a hymn about peace and justice, stopped my mind from wandering and distracted me from thinking about my own fears. Every single word of the prayer seemed to make a statement to me. I wanted the world to hear its message too.

Make me a channel of your peace.
Where there is hatred let me bring your love;
Where there is injury your pardon, God;
And where there's doubt, true faith in you.

Oh, Master grant that I may never seek
So much to be consoled as to console;
To be understood as to understand;
To be loved as to love with all my soul.
Make me a channel of your peace.
Where there's despair in life let me bring hope;
Where there is darkness, only light;
And where there's sadness, ever joy.

I prayed a lot after 9/11. I didn't really get where God fitted in with all this, or even where he fitted into my life anymore, but I still believed that having a faith, no matter which one, gives strength.

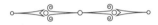

For the next four months or so New Yorkers hibernated. Couples stayed home safe in each other's arms, families cradled their children to sleep and single New Yorkers, like me, stayed home alone. We looked at the four walls and faced our fears as best we could. The mood of the city had changed and people had no interest in going out. I thought about my fears, my goals, my dreams, my hopes, my loves—my life. Night after night I looked through my tiny apartment window across to the United Nations, still saddened by the sight of the rooftop SWAT teams and sanitation trucks. I wondered how the world had come to this and whether New York was the place for me. Mum wanted me to come home, Steve told me I had a job to do and that I should stay. He was right.

In some ways I *did* want to run home to Australia but 'my kids' needed me. It wasn't enough to have guided them through September 11, they needed me for the whole year. They sensed turmoil in their world even if they didn't know why. They needed the security of knowing that school was a safe haven. If their teacher ran away, the sanctity of their world would have been threatened again. I simply could not do that.

In an email to my girlfriends in Australia I wrote:

25 October 2001

Hi Girls, finally I feel like writing again. It has been too hard to think about things too deeply till now. It was just easier to block it all out. But I am getting so many questions from my friends that I feel it's time to talk.

Since September 11 my life has changed. It has made me re-evaluate the true meaning of life and the value of friendships and family. It has also forced me to contemplate the harshness of the world, and though I have not suffered a personal loss I have been a witness to the terror, the fear of the unknown and the anxiety of not knowing when it will all stop.

Life since then has not been the same and probably never will be. This city has earned a special place in my heart and I feel so sad for New York. It will be decades before 'she' recovers. Most noticeable is the change in pace. There are less people, less energy in the streets, less laughter and a heavy heartedness.

The biggest pain and greatest challenge for me has been with my class. I rocked and cradled kids in my arms for two weeks after the attacks. There are still many tears. The kids don't really know why they are crying. They think it's because of their broken pencil, but I know better.

So what is the new normal? I have mostly sleepless nights and constantly wonder 'what's going to happen today?' I avoid the subway and the sight of rifle-bearing National Guards at Grand Central station freaks me out. I watch others with suspicion if I venture out for fear of a suicide bombing and think twice before I go where there are crowds. It's all about self-preservation right now.

I am also really 'pissed off' because I worked damn hard to get myself here and all of a sudden the place as I know it is gone. It will never to be the same again.

Guts it out? Yeah I reckon. For how long? Don't know. Live life to the fullest? Now more than ever.

So know that I 'love ya'.

I want you to go out and live a lot and love a lot too.

God bless

Kaz x

Dad stayed for one month while I recovered from 9/11. He kept me company and changed my disgusting 'new' studio into a livable space with paint, new carpet and windows. He did an amazing job—but I still couldn't get past the fact that I was living in a tiny rectangle of an apartment, in a city under threat while waiting for my now missing furniture to arrive from Australia. The transport company had gone bankrupt and my most precious belongings and photos were lost in transit.

So there we were, dad and me, eating and sitting on the floor, sleeping on mattresses on the floor in stressful New York City. It wasn't quite the dream I had played out in my mind. It wasn't supposed to be like this. But my disease had taught me to be resilient. I just had to dig deeper because I wasn't leaving NYC and I wasn't leaving 'my kids'.

Chapter 16
By Your Side

When Charlotte invited me to her wedding in the autumn of 2000, I happily accepted, I didn't know that night that I had met the man I would marry three years later—Charlotte's brother, Matthew.

It was not love at first sight. For starters, I was almost ten years older than Matt. And then there was the little matter of my crippling disease. Maybe because he seemed way too young for me and maybe because Charlotte had told me, later, that he'd developed a puppyish crush on me, Matt was the first man I told straight off the hard facts of RA's devastation.

The deaths of Matthew and Charlotte's parents—8 weeks apart—rocked their family. Having met me and heard something of my wonderful homeland, he chose to go to Australia to get over his grief. His friends had learned not to ask too many questions and knew to just let him go, so did Charlotte. Matt felt relief Down Under for the first time since the death of his parents. 'It was fun—happy people; people in England aren't like that,' he said

He returned home and Charlotte, who was still suffering from deep grief, again asked me to contact Matthew. It was a few months after his trip and he was still unsettled. As one of the few people at work who knew about my struggles with RA, Charlotte thought I might be able to help her brother wrestle with the enormity of what he'd just been through.

Once I made contact with Matt, a lively exchange of emails followed. In June 2002, he arrived in New York for a holiday. Charlotte wanted to see her brother before her baby was born, but because she was heavily pregnant she wasn't much fun in the evenings. I agreed to take Matthew out one night to give him a break from the baby talk.

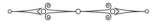

Matthew's facial features are sharp, perfectly defined and 'boyish'. His baby-blue eyes demanded attention—but perhaps that was because when you looked a little deeper you saw sadness. Matt had taken time off work in the London borough of Camden where he was an urban forester. His job involved protecting the English capital's Victorian tree population from harm and also helping in the restoration of historical garden squares.

We stopped on our first night out at an Irish Pub downtown in SoHo. It was packed. We stood at the 12 m (40-foot) long, dark wood bar as the World Cup Soccer streamed live from Korea in the background. I shifted the weight on and off my 'bad hip' as Matt and I chatted. He didn't notice. The bar had been an old car servicing garage and still kept the dirty cavernous feel.

With no warning, Matthew sheepishly asked: 'What would you do if I asked if I could kiss you right now?' I said: 'I'd say yes.' We kissed—passionately— at the bar. It was better than good and far nicer than I had expected. I wasn't into public displays of affection so we knocked it on the head at 3 a.m. and grabbed a cab back uptown.

I was flying to Australia the next day. It was the end of the academic year so I was headed home for some 'r and r'. I knew I needed to get some sleep. Timidly I escorted Matthew past my building's doorman. He gave me a disapproving nod and frowned as I pressed the UP button on the elevator. Matt and I stood waiting for it to transport us away from the censure zone.

Once we were in my apartment there was no holding back our passion. It was the first time we'd been naked together. He was gentle, loving, slow and adoring. I felt an attraction for him that I didn't anticipate. It was like I was being held by the right man for the very first time in my life. We didn't make love, but we both knew what we shared was different—there was such a close connection.

'What's that?' He pointed to the large scar on my right hip. I didn't lie and say it was a 'shark bite' as I'd always done before, particularly when I was asked on the beach. I felt compelled to be honest with Matthew.

'Hip-replacement surgery,' I said. 'I had it when I was about your age.'

Matt's reply made me feel less self-conscious. He said: 'I always think scars tell people's stories and the courage they've had in the past. Think of it as your badge of courage.'

The next day was a warm June, New York, Sunday morning. Matt and I walked past the Tudor City gardens to the corner of East 43rd and 2nd Avenues. As we kissed each other goodbye I caught a glimpse of the phone booth that I'd used to call Mum on 9/11. Things seemed a little better now.

My Qantas flight to Sydney was leaving in a few hours. With no plans to see each other again, Matthew returned home to Charlotte's apartment, pretending he'd escorted me home and fallen asleep on my couch. I thought about the night we'd shared over and over again on my long flight to Australia. I decided it wasn't likely to ever happen again. I told myself to dismiss it as just a bit of fun. And dismiss it I did, especially since I had work to do back in Oz.

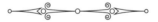

It baffled me that the biological medications that had given me so much relief in the US were not yet available in Australia. These included the Remicade infusion therapy that I'd received which works by correcting biological deviances—such as the immune system attacking itself—and blocking the cells that trigger inflammation. I understood that the unavailability of the 'biologics' in Australia was mostly due to their expense, but if people with arthritis could have access to these drugs then maybe they could get back into the workforce and save their bodies from further deformity and loss of mobility. That to me was a win–win situation. I wanted Australia to know that not only elderly people, but young people like me get arthritis—and that now they had reason to be optimistic and not so fearful. There was new hope.

It was time to 'claim my disease'. I was ready. Dealing with this illness and its devastation *quietly* was over for me. It was time to stand up and be a voice. This may not be the right course of action for all people who suffer from chronic disease, but it was right for me. After more than 20 years of hiding my pain and disability, I needed to unburden my secret. I wanted to end the deception and tell the world that even though I 'looked good', I wasn't. I was sick on the inside with a disease so aggressive that I hadn't had one pain-free day or night for years—until I found the new drugs.

Australians with arthritis living in my home country deserved the same opportunity. I felt a moral obligation to tell my story in the hope that the Government would see the urgent need to act and approve the biologics. I wanted Australians with arthritis to have access to the new medications that were available in the United States—and perhaps save them from hip or knee replacement surgery.

I felt so strongly about this that I decided to ring *Time* Australia magazine and tell them my story.

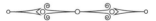

Multiple conversations, one interview and a photoshoot later, I had secured my first significant achievement as an advocate for sufferers of RA, arthritis, auto-immune diseases and chronic illness. My article was published in July 2002, just two weeks after I'd returned home to New York. The whole experience was fun, exciting, challenging and gave me a taste of what I could achieve if shared my story, through the media, with other sufferers. It was empowering. I had begun my journey as an arthritis advocate.

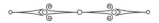

Matt had no intention of dismissing the memory of our night together as I had. He pursued me. He felt a stronger connection than I had experienced. Our journeys had been very different, but the same things seemed to bond us—bravery, courage and love. London called me. I called London. Email tripped over email. Our transatlantic love affair blossomed.

Email from Matt: Sunday, 1 July 2002

Dear Karen,

I am now back in the Big Smoke (London) and sitting at my desk considering what to do with the 415 e-mails in my inbox. It is tempting to perform a select all and delete exercise using only three fingers, or I could read them. Perhaps I need to flip the coin of fate to decide this tricky issue.

I had an excellent two weeks in NY and I am really proud of my sister with her big tummy. The Hamptons was totally not how it was 'supposed to be' and I think I prefer the European beach resorts with bars/beach and beach house together rather than driving in large 4WDs the whole time to get around. It was very relaxing though and my Celtic skin nearly tanned—but then decided not to. That's the trouble with using factor 30 paint as suntan cream. Thanks for taking me out, as I had a fantastic night. Not only are you great, but you also drink neat tequila—can't keep a good woman down. Your apartment is dead cool and waking up with you was just the best. I am just sorry the morning didn't last longer. Did I snore? How often do you meet a man with toothpaste all around his mouth? When I arrived back home to my sister's that morning they just assumed I slept on the sofa, so I kind of left it at that. I did tell them I had a big crush on you though. Anyway, I would love to see you again when you are in London at the end of next month but that's up to you. No pressure. E-mail me if you want to go out, I know you have some mates to catch up with as well so only if you have time. So just let me know.

Hope to see you soon and please don't worry about me.

Love Matt

PS Thanks for my World Cup Soccer handkerchief and you can stay at my place in London, of course, whatever happens.

My response to Matthew was brief. I committed to catching up with him and having some fun as friends. I was now holidaying in Europe on a farm in the south of France with my family because Steve had been completing Airbus training in Toulouse. I would be passing through London during the summer but was adamant that I would stay with my Australian girlfriend and told myself that it was ridiculous to entertain any ideas of a relationship with Matt. After all, he lived in London, was ten years younger than me and was the little brother of one of my best friends in NY.

Email from Matt: Wednesday, 10 July 2002

Dear Karen,

I know you have other people/places to see when you are in London so just tell me how you want to play it. We could do a Thursday night (restaurant), Friday day (sightseeing) thing as I expect you will be going out with your friends on the last night. I am not sure how you want to spend your holiday so you tell me as I am up for anything where you are concerned.

It will be so good to see you again.

Take care and speak to you soon.

Love Matt xxx

Email from Matt: Tuesday, 20 August 2002

Dear Karen,

All you need to know is that coming to the airport to see you is all I want to do and all I have been thinking about doing for some time. As long as you're there then that's all that matters. I would love for you to come back into town for a night, but as you have been on the Euro trail for four weeks it is always nice to get home; so you tell me. I know you are independent and like being dead tough in these sort of situations due to past experiences. I guess we are both a bit battle weary and it is hard sometimes to actually work out what is going on under everything else. Being with you feels good to me and it's where I want to be. Who knows what is around the corner? See you at Heathrow Terminal 1. You take care now.

Love Matt

I had decided that I needed to catch up with Matt—mainly to see if I still felt he was so special to me. When I landed at Heathrow he was waiting outside the arrivals gate at Terminal One. I'd been shopping in France for a new outfit to wear. It was a light blue

215

floral dress which sat just off the shoulders drawing attention to my bust, but in an innocent 'school girl' type of way. The hem fell well below my knees and the dress fitted snuggly over the rest of my 1.8 m (6 foot) frame. Wearing it made me feel special because it was new. I hung back before I walked through the arrival doors and dabbed some gloss on my lips. Little nervous pangs were darting around in my stomach. 'Don't be ridiculous,' I told myself. 'Get a grip, Kaz.'

I spied Matt first. He was standing nervously, both hands in his jean pockets, waiting with a black and red messenger bag slung over one shoulder. When he saw me he walked straight over and wrapped his arms around my waist. I bowed my head and sheepishly half hugged and half patted him on the back as he said: 'It's really good to see you.'

We caught the Heathrow Express into Paddington and then the Tube to my girlfriend Cheryl's place in Earl's Court. Cheryl lived in a large apartment. It was a typical London Georgian terrace. I'd met her and her husband, Al, in New York. They were Aussie expats and had moved across the Atlantic for work. I couldn't wait to see Cheryl; she was part of the attraction of London. We always had a laugh together.

As Matt and I sat hand in hand on the Tube I wondered if he was feeling the same heart flutters that I was. He had taken Friday off work and would be back to pick me up in the morning. He planned to play the tourist guide and show me around London. Cheryl suggested with a smirk that I pack my toothbrush in my handbag just in case 'day turned into night'.

Matt took me to the Tate Modern and we returned to the north bank of the River Thames via the Millennium Bridge. Halfway over the bridge we stopped and looked across the river towards the dome of St Paul's Cathedral. I wanted to be careful and guard my feelings, but I knew that Matt boosted my energy levels. Happiness was spilling from him into me. Day did turn into night and my feelings grew stronger.

Email from Matt: Wednesday, 28 August 2002

Morning Kaz,

Just a rapid hello and a kiss on the cheek on your first day back to work after a long hot summer. I loved seeing you in London. Thanks for making the effort to stopover on your way home to NY.

MPWxxxxxxxxxxxxxxxxxxxxxxxxx

Transatlantic emails flew almost daily in a fast and furious way. I told Matt all about my work, my social activities and hinted about how I felt about him. If I came home at night and there wasn't an email from him I felt disappointed. We slipped into using our nicknames—he was Matto, I was Kaz or a dozen variations on that theme including Kazbar, Kazarina, Kazabanka or plain Kazza. There was a surface lightness to our correspondence with an undercurrent of romance that was moving inexorably towards commitment. The courtship was unlike anything I had known before and I felt as if I was on cloud nine.

Email from Matt: Monday, 2 September 2002

Please fall in love with me.

Email to Matt, Monday, 2 September 2002

I am !!!!!!!!xxxxxxxxxxxxxxxxxxxxxxxxxxxxxxxxxxxxxxxxxxxxxxxxxxxx

In our emails Matt talked to me about the trouble he was having in coming to terms with his parents' deaths and I shared my fears about RA—but joyfully reported that I was in remission because of the new biological drugs. He knew that I hadn't felt so good for 20 years and responded by sharing with me the wit and wisdom of Oscar Wilde: 'We are all in the gutter, but some of us are looking at the stars.' Already Matt was planning a visit to New York to see me.

Every little thing that happened to me was of vital importance to him. News that I had undergone blood tests which confirmed my clinical remission brought this emailed response:

Dear Kaz,

When I am in NYC I would like to do something to celebrate your excellent blood test results. I know people easily forget news like that because they are not immediately attached to it, or find it difficult to understand. Of course it is a massive deal for you and I would like to be with you to mark it as an important and positive time.

Clinical remission really means that your disease is under control, honey, and even though that is because of the medication you still need to celebrate this.

Let me know what you think.

Love Mattoxxxxxx

On the first anniversary of 9/11 I wrote to him saying that I was strangely okay—it was the Monday preceding it which was the worst. On that day I had been anticipating the mourning and sadness that would come flooding back and began feeling quite depressed. On the day of the anniversary I attended the Australian American Memorial Service and started to feel that it was now time to use the pain as a platform from which I could move on. After a year of mourning it was time to reflect and put some of the pain behind us.

I shared the news of our romance with Charlotte and her husband, Eric, now the very proud parents of Peter who had been named after Charlotte and Matt's father. She was delighted that Matt and I had become an 'item' and I could see that wedding bells were in her mind's eye.

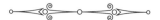

My efforts at highlighting the plight of sufferers of RA in Sydney had not gone unnoticed. A few days after the 9/11 anniversary I had a telephone interview with a political reporter, Mark Metherell from the *Sydney Morning Herald*. It was a milestone in my attempt to become a 'voice' for sufferers of arthritis in Australia and to get the Australian Government to add the wonderful new drugs that put me into clinical remission—after years of pain—on the pharmaceutical benefits list.

Not long afterwards I was honoured to receive an email from the chief executive of the Australian Arthritis Foundation. She thanked me for my work in generating publicity around the need for the new drugs.

By the end of 2003 a number of biological medicines, including Remicade, had regulatory approval on the Australian pharmaceutical benefits list. This meant that those suffering from RA, Crohns, psoriasis and other chronic diseases had access to 'miracle drugs' which were previously not affordable to the average patient. They cost more than A$15,000 per year of treatment.

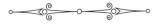

The thought of having a visit from Matt was a great motivator. I worked on my apartment until it shone and, for the first time in my life, went to a gymnasium to work out. I wanted to be as fit as I could possibly be for his visit—and his support for me and the lobbying work I was doing for RA sufferers never wavered.

Email from Matt: Monday,16 September 2002

Dear Kazbar,

Well done, honey, great work for an important cause.

Did you know I am seeing you next week? Sounds good doesn't it? I just can't wait to be with you again. I keep telling people about my Australian girlfriend in New York City. I like saying that because for a split second I think of you and smile because I know I am a lucky man with a perfect woman. I so want you. I try to write straight from the heart, like my sis. I love the way you and my sis get on. She adores you and knows you are good for her younger bro.

Not only are you gorgeous, you are selfless in your pursuit of achieving goals. I am excited and scared about reading about you and RA in the Australian Time *magazine. Not only because it will start to make me understand what you have been through with your battle against rheumatoid arthritis, but also because I am scared I will feel inadequate compared to you. I totally respect you and your battles with the disease. Thanks for sending me a copy.*

I am falling for all of you in every way. I can't wait to hear your heart beat and to feel your body against mine.

Love Matto xxoo

Matt made a couple of fun trips across the Atlantic to spend time with me and, before we knew it, we were counting down the days to see each other for Christmas.

New York woke to a white Christmas that year. By noon the grey clouds had rolled in and the snow flurries had turned into a blizzard. It didn't dampen our spirits. I was happy and Matt seemed ready to build new memories after a couple of painful Christmases.

We came in late on Christmas night after lunch with Charlotte and Eric. We snuck past the night doorman who was asleep. At least this time I had Matt with me and I didn't have to wake the doorman up so he could pull off my boots.

It was during these holidays that Matt decided that he wanted to move to New York so that we could be together. However, he knew that I had been hurt by men in the past and that I had some issues to get straight about him arriving in NY and about the pace of our romance.

'We need to plan and work out our goals because I don't want a relationship that slows or stagnates,' he said in an email.

'We're both positive and proactive people and I know we'll both work very hard to have a dynamic and strong relationship.'

His last email from London—on 6 February 2003—let me know exactly how he felt.

Dear Honey,

I am imagining Sade and Coldplay playing in your apartment and drinking Aussie red wine. Looking forward to holding your hand and seeing you smile. I was thinking about you wearing your Tiffany Christmas Bracelet and that made me smile. Come on Friday and roll on the following Saturday. I will be so nervous just before I see you again—butterflies and all.

Missing you like mad. NYC here I finally come.

Love from YOUR lucky boyfriend

Matto xxx

PS Let's get naked soon and eat cheese in bed. Let's walk in Central Park and catch a movie on the way home. It's all good, honey! You are my one.

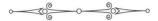

The RA didn't scare Matt off. He moved to New York and unpacked his life in my studio apartment. That autumn, on United Nations Day—a school holiday for those of us at the UN school—we were married at City Hall. Charlotte was our witness. We handed a camera to a passerby and posed for a snap in sunglasses and Cheshire grins.

I never thought about that day again because in my mind it didn't count. Our official ceremony was in Australia on American Independence Day, 4 July 2004, against a backdrop of the sparkling Sydney Harbour Bridge, balmy weather and the smiling Luna Park entry face.

Luna Park was a little reminder of New York for us because its name had its origins in Coney Island, a themed amusement park in metropolitan New York. As luck would have it a barge full of fireworks for a private explosives display was positioned on Sydney Harbour exactly between our venue, Aqua Dining, and another restaurant. As I sipped my champagne by the side of my husband I was sure the flutters of purple, yellow and pink lights in the night sky were signs of his parents' presence.

Everything was perfect on my wedding day. My dress was silver satin, much like the shade of the snow clouds on our first Christmas morning together. The halter neck and bodice were laced with Schwarzkopf crystals and the back plunged into a deep V around my hips. Steve, Trudy and their boys, Mum and Dad, Charlotte and Eric were with us. Father Mick, from our Black Rock days married us. Lisa was my bridesmaid, Venessa flew to Australia from New York, Dani, Margo and all the girls joined us for the celebration and my disease was under control. I couldn't ask for more. Mark Lizotte, my guest, generously sang a live version of Sade's *By Your Side* at the reception after I'd had four false starts at walking down the aisle because of a failing sound system at the quaint but antiquated Mercy College chapel.

Although it didn't occur to me at the time, I now think that the music broke down because I had made the decision to walk down the aisle with just my Dad. The wisdom of hindsight tells me that for all that Mum and I had been through, Mum, like the song says, should have been 'by my side' too.

My brother's speech filled the restaurant with sentiment. Then Matt delivered his speech, holding back tears:

> *Before I met Kaz, on the morning of my mother's death, I found a small golden angel which I have always kept. I now know that this was a sign because I think Kaz is that angel. I have been blessed that this brave, gorgeous woman with the unstoppable spirit is now my wife. She brings light to the darkest room, she gives endlessly with no expectation to receive, she understands that life is not always fair but rarely complains. She is an inspiration to me. She is my angel who I love completely. To be by her side, hold her hand and to travel through life together is the greatest honour. Thank you, darling. You are my special one.*

Together we bought a little piece of Midtown in Tudor City, complete with a terrace and gargoyles and our very own view of the Chrysler. And we settled in—he as the Director of Tree Preservation in NYC with the Parks Department, me at school.

And then, after all my years around other people's children, I finally decided that I wanted one of my own. I wanted my fairy tale to have a bundle-of-joy ending.

I was 42. I'd never been so focused in my life.

Chapter 17

Forever Young

The questions start in late September, when the back-to-school buzz gives way to routine. That's when the children take a good long look at me. They've already taken my measure as a teacher—from day one I've been given little skills tests, as this year's class clown angles for attention and this year's rebel stages mini-mutinies. After a couple of weeks my new students know what to expect from me and I come into sharper focus.

'Miss Ager?' says Justine, standing beside my desk as I mark her maths sheet. 'Did you hurt your fingers?' Shy Justine, with droopy striped tights, has chosen a private moment to speak her mind. 'Poor Miss Ager, I'm sorry.'

Ajay's bolder. While I'm at the whiteboard reviewing spelling words he calls out: 'Why do you point like *that*, Miss Ager? Why don't-cha point like *this*?'

Waving his index finger and grinning, Ajay steals the spotlight and then his mischief leaps around the room. Maddie and Abdul giggle, Mohammed and Zach begin fencing with pencils, Sam slides from his chair to the carpet and now Jasmine's wandering over to root about in her backpack for snacks.

I kneel beside Ajay. It's no accident that he's assigned a seat in the front of the classroom—alongside me. Quietly, I say: 'Is shouting out a question the right thing or the wrong thing to do, Ajay?'

His eyes meet mine. I can see he wants my approval. In Grade Two that's usually the case.

'The wrong thing,' he says.

'So how can you fix that?'

'By listening to you and raising my hand, Miss Ager.'

I raise my voice slightly as I stand, careful to shift my weight on to my stronger left side. 'Who would like to stretch out the sounds in the next word for us?' I ask, giving my feet a little shake the kids can't see to loosen my ankles. Jasmine, with a snack-filled baggie bulging from her pocket, enthusiastically pumping the air with her arm. I nod at her and she flies to my side to commandeer the pen.

'Good girl, now can you sound the word?'

'Y-e-s-t-er-d-ay; Yesterday,' Jasmine says proudly.

My crippled fingers are forgotten for now but not for long. I hold my left hand in the air motioning the class to stop. One of the fingers is permanently bent. The kids think I want them to mimic me. I look around the room waiting for silence. Instead I hear Sam, Zach and Maddie call out in unison: 'How do you do that?' They try to bend their ring fingers down on their 'stop sign' hand. Laughing, I ask them to put their hands in their laps and we try to move on.

Joseph's locks of curly hair frame his sweet face. The September mornings have been hard for him. He gets anxious saying goodbye to his mum and usually cries. His desk is near mine to make him feel secure and on top of it, bolt upright, sits a treasured classroom teddy and the *Blue Day Book* to make him smile. The book is filled with pages of funny animal photographs. Grumpy hippos, smooching puppies and penguins doing yoga are normally enough to trick him into smiling. Joseph has been listening to the conversation about Miss Ager's 'funny fingers' going on on either side of him. He's quieter than usual, sitting tilting his chair back on two legs while looking down at his desk. I can tell he is thinking about me.

'Time for music class, my friends. Please put away your spelling books and stand quietly behind your tables. How will I know you're ready, J2KA?'

'We'll be standing quietly,' says Maddie.

'Excellent, sweetheart.'

'Children, when you walk to music class please stay in one line. Let's play the quiet game on the way. I know you can do it, my friends.'

The kids are greeted enthusiastically by their music teacher,

Ms Chung. Joseph. hangs back a minute, waiting to steal a moment with me alone.

'Are you okay, Joseph?' I ask, straining to get down on both knees so I could look him in the eye.

'I didn't know about bad stuff when I was in pre-school. I think I know about your struggles. Why does this finger really always curve like that?' He said gently stroking it. 'Can you wiggle it? What happened to you, Miss Ager?'

I was shocked at Joseph's uncanny intuition. Most children in Grade Two think only of themselves. I took a deep breath and said: 'I don't want you worrying about Miss Ager. I used to play basketball and hurt my finger. That's all. I'm fine. Do you feel like going to music now?' He nodded yes in a measured way.

Joseph was happy with my answer that day.

I did think about his questions and wondered what he meant by the words: 'I know your struggles'. I'm not sure he even knew; perhaps it was just a feeling he had. Kids pick up on your energy just like dogs do and Joseph was an old soul. He read the situation perfectly. Later that year Joseph and his family asked if they could walk with me in the Arthritis Walk. He still walks every year. Joseph has raised thousands of dollars for the Arthritis Foundation and was a keynote speaker to launch the event in 2008.

As I stood outside the music room that day I did feel sorry for myself in that dot of time. Flashing through my mind was the number of questions I'd been asked about my 'hurt fingers' by the children and the innumerable occasions I'd brushed off the comments of seven-year-olds like: 'Miss Ager's going to die soon because of her fingers.'

How did I hurt my fingers? I guess it was more like my fingers hurt me. My fingers, wrists, elbows, shoulders, hips, knees, ankles and my feet.

The great thing about children is that they don't allow you to feel sorry for yourself for long; that's one reason why I love them and love to teach.

'Miss Ager?'

I look down at Justine's tousled head. We're standing together in the school lobby at the end of a long day. It's pick-up time. Her nanny's late.

I study her serious face and brush a loose strand of hair from her forehead with my crippled hand. 'Yes, darling?'

She slips her arms around my waist. 'I love you,' she says. I feel better straightaway.

Looking up from my attendance book the next day my attention turns to Ahmed who was looking stressed,

'Good morning Ahmed, how are you feeling today?'

'Good morning, Miss Ager. I'm good.'

'How was your evening and your morning, Ahmed?'

'Well my brother was crying a lot and then a pipe broke and water went everywhere.'

'Aaaha,' I thought, 'that's exactly why I ask these questions each day.' I had sensed Ahmed was anxious. Now I knew that I couldn't expect him to settle into his schoolwork until he calmed his emotions. I'd have to pay him special attention today.

'Pedro, how are you, darling?'

'I'm good because I have soccer this afternoon.'

'Justine, how are you feeling today?'

No reply. I repeat the question.

Justine is gazing out the window. 'Miss Ager, why don't you have kids? You got married. My, my, my dad can get you one from Africa to not make you sad.'

The chatter continues. Zach wriggles on the floor and decides it's his turn to comment.

'You need special things in a man to make a baby. It takes a long time with your husband. My bio dad (biological father) donated his parts. I never met my bio dad and neither did my mum. It's like when you donate to the bank and you never see the money again.'

I was trying to refocus my class without showing a reaction, but there were butterflies in my stomach because their comments had been a little too 'close to home'. I quietly said, 'Justine, let's try again. How are you today?'

'I'm good. Mum's picking me up today so I'm happy.'

As I walked to get my morning coffee I considered that there were probably many parents who had stories to tell about the obstacles they'd faced to have their child. My journey was just beginning.

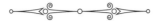

I did my research, as I've taught my students to do. I weighed the risks to my battle-scarred body, as I've done so many times before. Then I made my run at motherhood—beginning by switching to a RA syringe medicine thought to be safe for conception and on to fertility-drug injections, artificial inseminations, in-vitro fertilisations.

It was September 2006. I hurried through the school gates and flagged a cab. As the driver merged into traffic on the Franklin Roosevelt Drive, I sank deeper in the vinyl backseat. I was excited, a little nervous. I re-read a text message from my husband that had arrived at lunchtime: 'All done, babycakes. Good luck.' Shortly after I'd gotten Matt's message, I blurted to the school principal: 'I'm going uptown this afternoon to have an artificial insemination!'

It was blurted out to my childless principal—who briefly registered shock before rearranging her features into the cheery face she wore all day. The poor woman was trying to tell me about an upcoming meeting. There are always meetings to fill teachers' schedules at the beginning of the school year. I'd have to try to ingratiate myself at the one tomorrow—and keep my mouth shut about my extra-curriculars. But I could worry about that tomorrow. My appointment overshadowed other thoughts.

Good luck, Matt had wished for me—for us. He was part of my good luck.

Now, three years after I'd met him at Charlotte's wedding, we were more in sync than ever. As I got out of the cab at a hulking brick building in the East Nineties, I felt a giddy kind of happiness that I registered as inappropriate—dangerous, even—for a 42-year-old woman at the doorstep of a fertility clinic. A few weeks before I'd been there with Matt for a sit-down with the doctor to review our file and discuss my RA. I knew that my chances of conceiving and carrying a healthy baby were lower than for others of my age because of my immune system. RA's self-destructive programming might cause my body to launch an attack on a fertilised egg and prevent implantation. I knew the wild hormonal ride of pregnancy might pose special risks for me because of the way hormones interact with the multiple medicines I take to control my disease. And I knew my 33-year-old husband wasn't as keen on parenthood as I was—he was doing this because it was important to me. My desire for a child had become his desire to make me happy and that made me feel closer to him than ever before.

In some ways I was already on that wild hormonal ride. I'd been injecting myself in the belly, morning and night for two weeks, with medications to stimulate my ovaries. My stomach was hard in some places with marble-like balls which sat just below the surface of the skin. For all the effort I wasn't responding that well to the IVF drugs I'd been given to increase egg production.

I told the receptionist my name and took the one straight-backed chair among the overstuffed couches in the waiting room. I pictured Matt here earlier in the day and wondered what excuse he'd used to take a break from his Parks Department job in Brooklyn to come back to Manhattan and produce a test tube of sperm. For me. For us.

A lovely young woman with golden skin offset by her white lab coat called my name and I followed her to an examination room, where I shed my clothing below the waist and put on a green cotton gown. Waiting on the paper-lined table, I smiled at the memory of Matt and me leaving here together after our initial appointment last month, happy to have been told that tests of Matt's sperm showed them to be plentiful and 'mobile'—or good little swimmers and that I was responding well to the drugs I'd been given to increase egg production. We'd burst out the front door into the wet August air giggling like schoolchildren. Our new doctor, we'd decided, with his shiny bald head and plump features, looked like a life-sized version of the plastic bobblehead figurines on his desk.

Dr Horner arrived, with a test tube in his pudgy hand. 'Karen Ann Ager?' he said by way of greeting, as if we'd never met.

'That's me.'

He turned the test tube on its side to read the label. 'Matthew

Peter Wells,' he said, 'is that your husband's name?'

'Yes.'

'Very good. Let's begin.'

I wondered for a minute, in a silly, immature way, why I hadn't just tried the 'turkey baster' method using a large eye dropper at home. My ovulation had been triggered with another fertility medication and I was waiting to be injected with Matt's sperm. I lay back on the exam table after the doctor removed the catheter and waited for the quarter-hour prescribed, I felt closer to Matt than ever before. I had hope.

But our roller-coaster ride had only just begun. Every month there was new hope then it was dashed. Hope, no hope; hope, no hope. I'd get my period and the hope would be taken away until I started on the fertility drugs again. Each morning and night, Matt and I worked as a team as he mixed the meds for the syringes and I injected. We did back-to-back cycles for months and still no baby. I knew I didn't have much time left and my body was 'primed' so we had to keep going; there was no time to take even a month off. The doctors had done tests on my egg quality. I had seven months at best. The pressure was mounting. I didn't care what the drugs were doing to my body I just wanted a baby. The seven-month timeline was shocking news for me. But I had only myself to blame—I'd left it too long. Too influenced by Hollywood and its 40-something mums who were portrayed as the norm not the exception. I naively thought that a baby at 42 was typical—especially in New York.

Nine months later, thousands of American dollars worth of fertility drugs, three embryos and three failed implantations and Matt was gone.

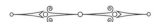

Nine months. That must be the punch line. I haven't figured out the joke.

I did my research but couldn't get pregnant, I weighed the risks to my body but not to my marriage. Did my husband leave because I couldn't have a kid or because I wanted one? Was it our age difference? Lack of communication? The stress and expense of fertility treatments?

Did it matter? Of course it mattered. I had to figure out a way of understanding this chaos. For a while I felt that by pushing Matt to do cycle after cycle I'd tipped our marriage over the edge. I blamed myself for his distress. It was just three weeks after our last attempt when he told me he was leaving. Wasn't the decision to have a family supposed to be a time when we felt closer than ever? After all we were trying to conceive our baby together. But I'd been on the IVF treadmill and I didn't see for a second that my husband was detaching. I never even stopped to wonder why he didn't want to make love to me anymore.

The Sunday he announced he was leaving I was shocked and hurt to the depths of my being. I didn't want to be anywhere near him; it was too painful. But in our 550 square foot New York apartment there was nowhere to go. So I did what fighting New Yorkers do; I walked the streets, I sat in Starbucks, I escaped to my cupboard or found some other retreat elsewhere in the apartment like the bathroom. Crying inconsolably, I succumbed to despair and let my limp body slide down the white tiled bathroom wall on to the floor. This was my 'bathroom floor moment', as Oprah likes to call it. I was in utter disbelief about my new reality. I'd never felt this type of pain and I had no idea how I was ever going to cope. I knew I'd need to call on a different type of strength than it had taken to fight my RA.

So I prayed.

But I didn't pray to God. I prayed to Matt's mum and dad. I asked them to somehow get us through this and to give me a sign that we'd be okay. Every Sunday night Matt and I would say 'hi' to them while lying in bed and we'd tell them about our week. Now it was just me praying; but I needed their help. The sign came a few days after Matt had left. He text me to see if I was okay and I detected a shift in his tone. It was entirely different to the man who had sat emotionless and completely disconnected in the lounge room while I was crying alone in the bathroom. The text didn't take away my pain but it made me feel calmer, more peaceful and somehow like my prayers had been answered.

Matt's message also gave me the strength I needed to deliver a promised speech for the Arthritis Foundation, paradoxically about resilience and how to cope—not, of course with the sudden and devastating end of a marriage, but with RA.

Looking back, in the cold light of day, I knew that losing Matt was only part of my distress. I was still grieving for the baby I never had. I looked at pregnant women enviously as I walked along the streets of Manhattan.

A few weeks after Matt left I put all my expensive fertility drugs into a bag and jumped into a New York cab to the IVF clinic to donate them, hoping they would help some other unfortunate childless couple achieve their dream. As I sat at the lights on East 69th Street and Park Avenue, a curly-haired lady about my age crossed the street. She was probably eight months pregnant. I wept. Shortly after I closed the door on the possibility of motherhood and sought professional help to guide me through my grief. I learnt to acknowledge that to have tried IVF for months and to have failed is a legitimate loss. And it's a loss for Matt too. That's why I wasn't angry with him, but I was still immeasurably sad. We'd run out of time. My heart was aching for the child that we would never have. My biggest wish was for 'just one more day', just a little more time. Perhaps there is nothing sadder in the world than running out of time.

Matt moved in with Charlotte and Eric. I felt like I'd lost them too. It wasn't that Charlotte wasn't there for me; she was and our friendship rose above the pain. But I thought about the dinners and the wine and the family support that Matt had when I was all alone. It hurt.

I didn't tell my own family that Matt and I had separated for more than a month. I didn't want them to think less of him. Not telling them isolated me even more. But one of my dearest friends was there.

A few days after Matt moved out Venessa rang. I was in tears when I answered the phone and in between sobs said: 'Matt's left me; he's gone.'

'I'll be there in 20 minutes,' she said as she dropped the phone.

Her BMW powered along Franklin Roosevelt Drive, the pelting rain hitting the windscreen as she made her way to midtown.

Venessa is what we Aussies call salt of the earth. She doesn't judge, is loyal and never expects anything in return. She gave me the strength to get through the shock of my separation.

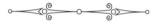

In the beginning I met with Matt once a week to talk. I was desperate to reconcile. Time and again I would say to him: 'Honey, I'm coming to you from a place of love and understanding. Please come home.' Opposite me sat a man who I didn't really know anymore. Somewhere in the chain of events between our wedding, the many adjustments he had to make to live with me in New York, artificial inseminations and IVF treatments I lost my husband.

'You didn't listen to me when I said I didn't really want kids and I had to look at my wife with bruises all over her stomach practically killing herself to have a baby,' he said.

Listening skills—I taught them every day and judged how my little charges were accepting and adopting them. But I'd failed to make the grade myself. I had sleepless nights for months. After going to bed I would fall into a deep sleep, but in the wee hours of the morning I'd be wide awake, staring through the translucent blind at the lights of the Chrysler Building. The long dark nights were the loneliest in my life. I'd will myself to get through them with the same internal voice I had used when I was desperately sick with RA saying: 'C'mon, Kaz, be strong. What's one action you can do to get yourself out of this moment?' Usually the answer was simple. I'd pick up a book or call Australia. Lisa and a few other friends knew Matt had left by now. It was daytime in Oz so they could talk me through my late night loneliness.

At work I walked around wearing a fixed smile. In actuality it was a mask behind which I hid. But the children, a few colleagues and my teaching career were my saving grace. The kids were always ready to give me a hug, or make me laugh through their straight-forward questioning and unforgettable insight. They're wise—so much wiser than their six or seven years. In the course of a day I'd come to expect at least a few memorable one-liners that would provide instant cheer.

'Good news softens you up and bad news breaks you down.'

'The life lesson I learned today is that if you ignore hurtful words you always win.'

'Your Dad's 73, Miss Ager! Wow, how did he last that long?'

'My Dad's bald, I think my Dad's hair fell from his head onto his back.'

'A good person tries new things, like trying a new ice-cream. At least try a new taste! Sometimes you have to do things you don't like. I want you to like new things. It's simple. I'm not telling you to eat vanilla. I am just suggesting it.'

'Red is one of the rarest moustaches.'

'Girls play Barbies.' 'No we don't. You could search my house for one and you wouldn't find one.'

'My brother likes Barbie girls because he thinks when you have a girlfriend you have to like what they like.'

'Your parents are separated. That's sad. Did you get a stepdad yet? I hope not cause then I'll feel really bad for you.'

'Sshh, it's none of your business.'

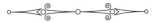

The kids helped to get me through my darkest days until I told my family. So did Dad's humorous telephone messages, which he left, ignorant of what was going on in my life.

'Hi, Max here, I mean Dad. I've just seen something about stray dogs on TV. If you meet one try to approach it from the side and never look into its eyes. Love you. Bye.'

A month after Matt left I told my family. Mum flew to New York within days of hearing the news. She was there for me again. My family saw it as a crisis and sent Mum over just like when they sent Dad after 9/11. Together Mum and I searched for answers. She stayed nearly 14 days. When she left all I had to do was 'hang in there' for a few weeks until my summer break. As soon as school was out I'd be on that Qantas silver bird again and home where I belonged at the moment.

Eight months after Matt left he stood in 'our bedroom', the Chrysler Building sparkling in the background, as I besieged him with questions about how he felt.

'I don't know how I feel. I've felt numb for six years. Since my Mum and Dad died I haven't been able to feel anything much.'

He was packing the last of his things to move to his new rental in Brooklyn. It was all too real now.

At that point I understood that I had had an emotionally detached husband for most of our marriage. I guess it is what happens to many couples. The daily grind, coupled with triggers from the past, and one or two other stressful situations and before you know it your marriage is in dire straits. That's what happened to us and I didn't see any of it coming. But the signs were there all along. I just didn't see them.

I think some men feel suffocated by the responsibilities of marriage and when they get 'maxed out' it's 'fight or flight'. Right or wrong, weak or strong—once men become emotionally detached I think there is no alternative for a woman other than to surrender. I'm not sure anymore what the commitment of marriage means because whether you're married or not, if a man decides he is leaving there's not a thing you can do to make them stay, or to get them back. Once I understood that and accepted it I could start the healing process.

After Matt left my Dad gave me some advice,

'Karen, the way you behave now will determine a lot.' He was right.

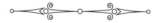

In the months following our separation I tried to understand my husband's pain rather than slip into the role of being a martyr. I understood that Matt never really gave himself permission to *stop grieving* for his parents. Our marriage and the IVF were attempts by Matt to move forward with his life. But he hadn't addressed his grief. Putting myself in his shoes diffused the anger I might have felt and enabled me to forgive him.

I imagined how hard it must have been for Matt to watch his parents in pain; to clean his mother's handbag out of all the things she thought she'd use again because she didn't expect to die; to see his Dad grieving for his wife; to meet and fall in love with his *special one* only to find out that she has a chronic disease which has the potential to take her from him; to shut the door on his family, friends and job in London and move countries; to try unsuccessfully to have a baby and to face a life of being childless. The string of losses in Matt's life added up and all contributed to the disaster that beset us.

During the time after my separation and throughout the healing process I learned a lot. I thought my life lessons were mostly to do with RA, but I was wrong. I began to understand that there are 'layers' to people's happiness and pain. With Matt there was his grief, then there was fear about me carrying a baby and then, after all the effort, there was the feeling of failure after months of trying for a child. There's a common thread in each layer. It was loss and fear of loss. Once I understood these things I stopped seeing myself as the victim and stopped blaming. In fact we both feared the same thing—abandonment.

About four months after Matt had moved to Brooklyn and after all our legal separation paperwork was final he called me. By now I was getting closer to accepting all that had happened. I was working on my role in the marriage breakdown with a professional and I wasn't 'needy' anymore. We hadn't been in regular communication for a while. During the phone call he asked: 'Would you please come to dinner with me to celebrate my birthday?'

'Okay, I guess so.'

Our time apart had meant soul-searching for us both.

Matt had booked a table for two in an area he knew I adored, Gramercy. It's filled with quaint, brick apartment buildings and has a village atmosphere. The restaurant had low, red velvet sofa-like chairs and French tea-party tables and, with its open fireplace, was warm and welcoming.

It was good to see him. Matt looked tired to me, thinner in the face and sad. When our eyes met across the candlelit table I felt like I'd missed him. I could see he'd missed me. There was more loss in his eyes. He took my hand and held it across the table.

'Babycakes, I am so sorry I disappointed you. I didn't mean to hurt you or your family.'

My eyes welled up with tears. When I heard these words I felt vindicated. I had no reply. I couldn't say 'it's okay' because that wasn't the truth, because none of this had been okay. But I listened. By listening, I knew Matt would feel I was giving him a chance at being understood.

By the end of the night we were having fun, like the old days. We had a few shots with the barman who shared the same birthday as Matt. Simplifying things, getting back to enjoying ourselves together and being present with each other was what we needed to do. Ipods, Blackberries and computers were all put away for the night. I could feel that Matt was trying to reconnect.

After that initial post-separation outing we began to go on occasional dates and started to remember why we fell in love. One night he said to me about our separation: 'Honey, I feel like I'm in this so deep now I don't know how to get out of it.' Then he told me he wanted to come home.

As much as I loved him I knew that I couldn't let this happen until I'd seen some consistent changes in how he behaved. I told him I needed hope, security and commitment in my life.

'For us to have a chance I need you to show me these things in your actions because right now I still can't believe your words.'

It was all part of the process.

Matt began weekly grief therapy sessions and recommitted to me financially, which gave me the hope that we were moving forward as a couple.

Seven months later he sub-leased his apartment in Brooklyn and moved back into our apartment. It was a short step to welcoming Willy into our home. Willy is our Morkie puppy dog, our very own bundle of joy. He looks like a little bear with soft silver fur, cream paws and a permanent smile on his little cheery face. He's a scruffy mix of Yorkshire Terrier and Maltese. Matt and I found his picture on the internet at the exact same time and then flew him to New York from Wisconsin. His price had been reduced because he was already four months old and I guess, the runt of the litter; all his brothers and sisters had been snapped up by pet-hungry families. When Matt picked him up from La Guardia airport he sat timidly in the back of the crate looking at his new 'Daddy', not knowing that he was about to become a New York pooch.

Willy Wells is named after a pug dog in *East Enders*, a well-known English soap opera which is set in a working-class, dockland area of London. One of the original characters was an old lady called Ethel who went everywhere with her little pug called Willy. Whenever Ethel's back was turned Willy would be into mischief. Her famous tagline was 'Oh Willy', which she would say as he performed another little naughty deed.

For the entire first night Willy sat bolt upright and peered through the grill of the wooden gate that separated him from Matt and me. He didn't take his eyes off the bedroom and I don't think I took my eyes off him either.

Little Willy had a gagging cough which worried me greatly. As I lay in bed looking at him and listening out for him I imagined the first night with a new-born baby and how frightened and on edge new parents must feel. Matt took Willy to the vet the next morning and we discovered that he had not been very well looked after by the breeder. He had ear mites and kennel cough. We were both worried. We had this responsibility and we felt almost powerless. However, Willy recovered quickly and our house was filled with love again. Every day when I come home from work I have the healing love of my puppy when I walk through the door. His positive energy has lifted the whole family and attracts smiles from many sweet old New York ladies. He has helped to simplify what we enjoy doing. Willy is happy with his three-dollar pink squeaky pig and being with his new 'pack'—Matt and me. Willy and Matt have bonded deeply—they go everywhere together and are in tune with one another.

Part of Matt's financial recommitment to the marriage was that he purchased a holiday apartment for us in South Beach, Miami. Willy travels on the plane with us in my handbag and loves the freedom of the beach, which reminds me of home. He has helped to heal my aching heart that came with my infertility and has made us feel like a family. I love him so much and, in a strange way, feel that I owe him a good deal. He may be scruffy and funny, but there is no pooch more pampered than him in the whole of the Big Apple.

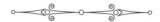

When I couldn't get pregnant I felt like my body was again refusing to cooperate with me just like it had snubbed me for all those years with my RA. I felt disappointed, even angry because, once again, it had let me down. I felt alienated by my own flesh and blood and utterly powerless in my quest for a child. But I knew there was a message in this pain somewhere, somehow. I just had to find it.

The first thing that I learnt was that I had to stop being so reckless with myself. Now that Matt was home I owed that to him. It was also time to be thankful for my body rather than angry with it. I admitted to myself that I had put it through hell over the years and it had kept on working. If I were an advocate for arthritis, I had to be an advocate for my own body too.

Somewhere, coded in my Australian DNA there must be a gene for getting on with things, come what may. My RA is once again active and the biological medicines are no longer controlling it so well, or preventing further joint damage. Some mornings I need long, hot showers to loosen my joints so I can go to work, a tradition I began in my teens, when I was thought to be suffering nothing more than growing pains. I have started to think of these recent flare-ups as my grown-up growing pains. While I know I can't beat RA, I've also proven it won't beat me.

So what else have I learned?

I think times of loss and despair are spiritual moments. They are moments when you become more open to contemplation, love and forgiveness. I think my little friend Amy knew a lot of this all those years ago. She knew life was sometimes not fair, but how she managed during her adversity was a measure of the person she was. It became a kind of yardstick for me—a benchmark above which I had to raise my chin. My disease had deformed my body but I'd fought for my spirit. My inability to conceive and the loss of my